GET WELL
LIVE WELL

A Guide to Living a Life of Health and Wholeness

Eva M. Francis

"In the beginning was the Word and the Word was with God and the Word was God."

— (John 1:1)

"Beloved, I wish above all things that thou mayest prosper and be in health, even as thy soul prospereth."— (3 John 1:2)

Discover the Secrets to Living a Life of Health and Wholeness

Eva M. Francis

HC, MSN, CCRN, NEA-BC

Except otherwise stated, all Bible references are from the King James Version.

ISBN: 9798346953418

Brilliant Healthcare Productions

15000 Pines Blvd, Suite 365,

Pembroke Pines, Florida 33029

Disclaimer

The Publisher and the Author make no representations or warranties with respect to the accuracy or completeness of the contents of this work. The information provided serves for educational and inspirational purposes only. No information included in this book should be used to treat or diagnose. Please contact your healthcare provider before making changes to your existing health regimen.

Dedication

To my beloved parents, Mrs. Eunice Francis and Mr. Vincent Francis, whose love and guidance shaped the person I am today. Your unwavering support and boundless encouragement inspired and shaped me to become who I am today. Though you are no longer with me, your legacy of love and your spirit lives on, in every word I write.

I dedicate this book to you, and my siblings with all my love.

Acknowledgments

This book, *Get Well, Live Well*, is about wholeness and reclaiming the health that God has given us. **It is God's divine will that we walk in health and wholeness. He never wants to see us walking in sickness and disease.**

I want to celebrate the individuals who have stood firmly on the Word of God and received their divine healing. I also want to acknowledge all the individuals who have prayed with me and encouraged me to dream big, helping me walk straight into my purpose. Let me take this moment to acknowledge my family's love and support, particularly my late parents, Mr. and Mrs. Vincent and Eunice Francis. I love you with all my heart.

I want to acknowledge the late Pastor Stan Moore, Sr., as well as Pastor Geri Moore from Words of Life Fellowship Church. They taught me how to "pray the Word, use the Word, and confess the Word." I love you so much and salute your wisdom, anointing, and biblical insights.

A heartfelt "thank you" to my sisters in Christ—Ingrid De Souza and Rose Reid—for assisting with the editing of this manuscript.

To all my family and friends who gave me permission to share their stories in this book, I love you.

Foreword

I can highly recommend this book with great confidence, not only because of its outstanding content but also because of the person who wrote it. I have known Eva Francis for over 27 years. Eva's lifelong ambition to see people get well and live well has been more than just a career; it has become a genuine calling. To describe how she has blessed my life would literally fill pages.

As a pastor, it has been my mission to touch every life I encounter. Every person is special in their own way, but occasionally, you meet someone who truly stands out from the crowd—someone who walks in the fullness of their gifts and calling and continually strives to help others live a better life. Eva M. Francis is one of those remarkable individuals, and I am blessed beyond measure to have her as part of my life.

As her pastor, I have had the great joy of watching Eva grow and mature in God's Word, living a life of love, compassion, commitment, and integrity. Thank you, Eva, for touching my life in such a profound way and for writing this powerful book to help others. I am certain that it will be a blessing to all who read it.

The late Pastor Stanley L. Moore Sr. Words of Life Fellowship Church, North Miami Beach, Florida

Why I Wrote This Book

With over 30 years of experience working as a registered nurse, I have seen how sick people have died helplessly just because they held onto the report they received from their doctors.

There is a power that supersedes the doctor's report and can turn things around. Yes, healthcare is beyond medications. However, there are lifestyle practices and Biblical Principles that, if followed, would elongate your life and also heal your diseases. This is what I will be sharing in this book.

God placed it on my heart to teach believers about health-related matters and how health and wellness are intertwined with God's Word. This book is written by the divine inspiration of the Holy Spirit.

Although I have worked with conventional medicine for over thirty years, God has taught me firsthand. Despite these decades, He is inspiring and allowing me to think outside the box when it comes to healing, health, and wellness.

God has shown me that living a healthy lifestyle is His will for us and He is ever ready to heal us whenever we are ill and restore our sound health. I have prayed for many patients and staff (at their request), and they received their healing. I have practical experience of the healing power of God and this is what I will be sharing with you in this book.

My response to individuals who ask my opinion on healing is that while physicians, nurses, and health professionals play a crucial role in promoting health, Jesus Christ is the true Healer. And I am sure that He will heal you as you read this book.

This book is not only scientifically based but spirit-filled, as my mission is to align medical science with what God says about our health and healing.

This book will be a life-changer for you. So, sit back, relax, and get ready to embark on a journey to another level in this season of your life. Be blessed as you navigate your inner being through the pages of this refreshing and anointed book.

How to Get the Most Out of This Book?

Because this book focuses on health, healing, wholeness, and claiming your body—your temple—I encourage you to read it prayerfully. Let every word and chapter penetrate your being as you seek to strengthen your physical and spiritual health. God promises us health, long life, wholeness, and soundness in His Word. As you read this book, reach out in faith and take hold of the health and wholeness that He has promised and provided.

Know that God has good health available for you. Understand that we should walk by faith—and not by fear. Many times, we believe in God's supernatural miracles for our lives, but when they don't manifest instantly, we can become discouraged and let fear creep in. We should counteract fear with the Word of God. When fear tries to come upon me, my first thought is this: "FALSE EVIDENCE, APPEARING REAL." It is not real, people. Let us crush it! Is this always an easy task? Absolutely not but it is surmountable!

Therefore, to get the most from this book, you must, first and foremost, be open-minded and realize that Jesus is both our Source and Healer.

When you have decided to be teachable, read, study, and meditate upon the words of this book thoroughly and prayerfully, expect Jesus Christ to open your heart and spirit to the shining light from heaven that brightens any dull areas of your health.

Be expectant; your health will be renewed, refreshed, and rejuvenated. You will experience God's power changing any health circumstances; this power is dynamic and will also impact you spiritually, emotionally, and financially. Trust God to do anything and everything for you. God is a God who changes things, people, and circumstances, and He will change your life.

A blood transfusion is important for an anemic individual, but I would say, "The Blood of Jesus Christ is far more important." To clarify, I am not suggesting that a blood transfusion is unnecessary; I am simply affirming that there is power in the blood of the Lamb. If your physician recommends a blood transfusion, I will say, "Take it," while also acknowledging and believing with all of your heart that the Blood of Jesus can heal you of that condition.

As you read through these pages about your health and healing, I know you will find hope. It is important to believe that God can and will heal. Yes, He will—if you only believe. If you are experiencing any ill health, just know that you have hope.

Speaking about the healing power of God, I have been healed of an ovarian cyst by the stripes of Jesus Christ, and I know, without a shadow of a doubt, that God is a Healer. He cares about our health, and He wants us to live a healthy and victorious life. He desires for us to reclaim our health and guard it with all our heart, mind, and spirit. Consider this as the work that God has assigned us to do.

We must be in the best shape of our bodies, spirit and minds to fulfill that calling and assignment.

I chose to write this book because so much information, knowledge, and wisdom have been deposited in me over the years by my parents, pastors, coaches, mentors, friends, family, and colleagues. I felt a divine inspiration to share this powerful message of health, wellness, hope, and healing, particularly with everyone who may read this book.

Many of us are accustomed to hearing these teachings from ministers, pastors, and apostles. However, I am reinforcing health and wellness through the application of lifestyle, science and Biblical Principles. I am passionate about giving back what I have learned over the years. I want to encourage every reader to be inspired by the pages of this book.

Take notes, LEARN, UNLEARN, and RELEARN. Let these teachings take root in your spirit, and you will see the manifestation of His glory. You will never be the same again. Get ready to call your friends and family to share new revelations. If you receive healing and are well again, call a friend and share the news. Encourage friends and family to read this book too.

Contents

Chapter 1

The Foundation of Health - Understanding the Basics

"Do you not know that your bodies are temples of the Holy Spirit, who is in you, whom you have received from God? You are not your own; you were bought at a price. Therefore, honor God with your bodies." - 1 Corinthians 6:19-20

According to the World Health Organization (WHO), health is defined as 'a state of complete physical, mental and social well-being and not merely the absence of disease or infirmity.' This definition emphasizes that health is not just about the absence of illness, but also includes a state of overall well-being in all aspects of a person's life.

Health is important for several reasons:

1. **Quality of Life:** Good health allows you to enjoy a high quality of life and engage in activities that bring you joy and fulfillment. When you are healthy, you can participate in work, leisure and social activities without limitations.

2. **Productivity:** Health is crucial for maintaining productivity in your personal and professional life. When you are healthy, you get better in being able to focus, concentrate and perform tasks effectively, leading to increased productivity.

3. **Prevention of Diseases:** Maintaining good health through healthy lifestyle choices such as proper nutrition, regular exercise and adequate rest can help prevent the onset of chronic diseases such as diabetes, heart disease, hypertension, obesity and certain types of cancer.

4. **Longevity:** Good health is closely linked to longevity. By taking care of your physical, mental and social well-being, you can increase your chances of living a longer and more fulfilling life.

5. **Emotional Well-being:** Health also plays a significant role in emotional well-being. When you are healthy, you are better equipped to handle stress, anxiety and other mental health challenges, leading to a greater sense of peace and contentment.

Understanding the Temple of the Holy Spirit

"Do you not know that your bodies are temples of the Holy Spirit, who is in you, whom you have received from God? You are not your own; you were bought at a price. Therefore, honor God with your bodies." - 1 Corinthians 6:19-20

The Bible teaches us that our bodies are temples of the Holy Spirit. This means that we are called to treat our bodies with respect and care, just as we would treat a sacred place of worship. By honoring our bodies, we are also honoring God, who created us in His image.

Physical Health

Taking care of our physical health is an important aspect of honoring God with our bodies. This includes eating a balanced diet, exercising regularly, getting enough rest and avoiding harmful substances.

Mental Health

Our mental health is just as important as our physical health. The Bible instructs us to renew our minds daily and to focus on things that are pure, lovely and of good report. By practicing gratitude, forgiveness and positive thinking, we can maintain our mental well-being and experience peace and joy in our lives.

Spiritual Health

Lastly, our spiritual health is crucial to our overall well-being. By spending time in prayer, reading the Bible and attending church, we can strengthen our relationship with God and grow in our faith. When we are spiritually healthy, we are better equipped to handle life's challenges and experience God's peace and presence in our lives.

Chapter 2

Nourishing Your Body God's Way

"Then God said, 'I give you every seed-bearing plant on the face of the whole earth and every tree that has fruit with seed in it. They will be yours for food." - Genesis 1:29

We live in a world where processed and unhealthy foods are glamorized and have become the day's order, even though they have severe health consequences. We have neglected and despised the natural and healthy foods God gave to us. To live well, you must be willing to make a change in this habit. However, you do not have to make a drastic change all at once. I believe that making changes one meal at a time is key to success in healthy living.

I remember years ago when I wanted to go the route of making a lifestyle change in my nutrition. I failed because I was trying to eliminate too many food items all at once. In the words of our late Pastor Stan Sr., "courage, commitment and consistency matter."

God wants us to eat the food He has created. There must be a reason why God requires us to eat the food He has provided. Eating God's natural foods and following a plant-based diet is a way of honoring our bodies and promoting our health and wellness. God has provided us with an abundance of natural foods that are meant to nourish and sustain life.

Fruits, vegetables, whole grains, nuts and seeds are all examples of God's creations that provide essential nutrients for our lives. By incorporating these foods into our diets, we can fuel our bodies with the vitamins, minerals and antioxidants needed for optimal health.

The Importance of Nutrition

Nutrition plays a vital role in maintaining good health and preventing disease. God's natural foods are rich in nutrients that support our immune system, aid in digestion and promote overall wellness. These plant-based foods can reduce our risk of chronic illnesses such as heart disease, diabetes and obesity. It is essential to prioritize nutrition and make conscious choices about what we put into our bodies.

Plant-Based Diet

A plant-based diet centers around eating whole, plant foods while minimizing or eliminating animal products. This dietary approach aligns with God's provision of natural foods and is associated with numerous health benefits. Plant-based foods are rich in fiber, vitamins, and antioxidants. This makes them an excellent choice for nourishing our body. Eating plant-based diets don't only improve our health but also protect the environment and show compassion for all of God's creations.

What the Bible Says About Eating Good Food

In Genesis 1:29, God gives us every *seed-bearing plant* and every tree with fruit for food, emphasizing the abundance of natural foods available to us. Proverbs 15:17 reminds us that it is better to eat vegetables with love than a fatted calf with hatred, highlighting the value of choosing wholesome foods with gratitude and compassion.

As a Jamaican, I appreciate the island's food culture, which is known for its bold and spicy flavors. Jamaican cuisine is influenced by a blend of African, European, and indigenous ingredients. Dishes like jerk chicken, ackee and salt fish, as well as rice and peas are staples in Jamaican households, reflecting the vibrant and diverse culinary heritage of the island.

While Jamaican food is undeniably delicious and satisfying, it is essential to consider the impact on our health when consumed regularly in large portions. Reflecting on my upbringing and the

5

foods I was raised with, I recognize that, while these dishes hold a special place in my heart, they may not always align with my health and wellness goals as I mature.

Wisdom and Moderation

While Jamaican cuisine is a cherished part of our cultural identity, it is crucial to approach it with moderation and mindfulness. Balancing traditional dishes with healthier alternatives and incorporating more plant-based options can help us enjoy the flavors of our heritage while nourishing our bodies in a way that promotes long-term health.

Here are some scriptures that emphasize the importance of eating healthily and treating our bodies as temples of the Holy Spirit:

1. **1 Corinthians 10:31** - *"So whether you eat or drink or whatever you do, do it all for the glory of God."*

2. **1 Corinthians 6:19-20** - *"Do you not know that your bodies are temples of the Holy Spirit, who is in you, whom you have received from God? You are not your own; you were bought at a price. Therefore, honor God with your body."*

3. **Genesis 1:29** - *"Then God said, 'I give you every seed-bearing plant on the face of the whole earth and every tree that has fruit with seed in it. They will be yours for food.'"*

4. **Proverbs 15:17** - *"Better a dish of vegetables with love than a fattened calf with hatred."*

5. **Daniel 1:12** - *"Please test your servants for ten days: Give us nothing but vegetables to eat and water to drink."*

These verses highlight the importance of honoring God with our food choices, treating our body as temples and nourishing ourselves with the provisions of the earth. By following these teachings, we can strive to eat healthily and live in alignment with God's will for our body.

Chapter 3

Moving Towards Wellness - The Role of Exercise and Physical Activity

"For bodily exercise profiteth little: but godliness is profitable unto all things, having promise of the life that now is, and of that which is to come." – 1Timothy 4:8

Movement and exercise play a crucial role in our overall wellness. Physical activity not only helps us maintain a healthy weight and prevent chronic diseases but also has a profound impact on our mental and emotional well-being. Regular exercise triggers the release of endorphins, often referred to as "feel-good" hormones, which help reduce stress, anxiety and depression, leaving us feeling happier and more content. Additionally, exercise has been shown to improve cognitive function and memory, making us sharper and more focused in our daily lives.

From a scientific perspective, movement and exercise are essential for maintaining a healthy cardiovascular system. Engaging in physical activity increases our heart rate, pumping oxygen-rich blood throughout our bodies and improving circulation. This not only strengthens the heart but also reduces the risk of developing cardiovascular diseases such as heart attacks and strokes.

Furthermore, regular exercise helps strengthen our muscles and bones, reducing our risk of injury and improving overall physical strength and endurance. This is especially important as we age, as maintaining muscle mass and bone density becomes crucial for preventing falls and fractures. Incorporating movement and exercise into our daily lives doesn't have to be complicated or time-consuming. Simple activities such as walking, biking, swimming or dancing can all have a positive impact on our health and well-being. Finding activities that we enjoy and can easily incorporate into our lifestyle is key to making exercise a sustainable habit.

Whether it's taking a daily walk around the neighborhood, joining a dance class or hitting the gym a few times a week, finding ways to stay active is essential for our overall wellness. By prioritizing movement and exercise in our lives, we can improve both our physical and mental health, leading to a happier and more fulfilling life. Remember, every step counts towards a healthier you.

Movement and exercise are not only important for our physical and mental well-being but also hold significance in a spiritual sense. "...You are not your own; you were bought at a price. Therefore, honor God with your bodies" (1 Corinthians 6:19-20). This verse underscores the importance of treating our bodies with respect and care, including engaging in activities that promote health and wellness.

Furthermore, the Bible emphasizes the benefits of physical activity and movement. In 1 Timothy 4:8, it states, "For physical training is of some value, but godliness has value for all things, holding promise for both the present life and the life to come." This verse reveals to us that while physical exercise is important, spiritual growth and godliness should also be prioritized in our lives.

As a Jamaican, we are known for excellence. As you may know, we are renowned for our excellence in track and field. At the time of this book's writing, Jamaica's pride, Usain Bolt holds the fastest record in 100 meters in the Olympics. Although I always wanted to be a runner, my parents prioritized academics. I didn't fully grasp the benefits of exercise, but as I grew older, I came to understand that any simple form of exercise is both safe and beneficial for the body. Exercise impacts not just physical health but also mental, emotional, relational and spiritual well-being.

8

Exercise ranks high among the essentials for good health and wellness. Other vital components include proper rest, hydration, fresh air and a balanced diet. Despite your New Year's resolutions, a lack of exercise remains a concern for families, friends and even governments.

Ten Reasons to Exercise

Many people need to follow an exercise program to maintain their health. You'll find below several compelling reasons to start exercising now. They include fat loss, disease prevention, an enhanced state of mind, enhanced relationships, added energy, boosted self-esteem, and improved thinking—all of these benefits contribute to a higher quality of life and can even reduce financial burdens related to health issues.

1. Bodily Exercises Contribute to Fat Loss

According to health experts, a poor diet and lack of exercise are major contributors to rising rates of certain diseases. Physical inactivity and being overweight are linked to premature deaths each year. Regular exercise is crucial for weight management; it helps to burn calories and when combined with a balanced diet, can lead to weight loss. Essentially, the more you exercise, the more calories you burn, which helps reduce body fat and manage weight. The key to effective weight loss is to ensure that you burn more calories through physical activity than you consume through nutrition.

2. Exercise Prevents and Treats Disease

Engaging in regular exercises has been shown to significantly reduce the risk of various diseases, including heart disease, cancer, diabetes and stroke. Exercise can also improve or even heal many of these conditions. Consistent exercise or a routine can lower HDL (High Density Lipoprotein) cholesterol levels, reduce triglyceride levels and decrease blood pressure. For men, regular physical activity lowers the risk of prostate cancer, while for women, it can reduce the risk of breast and uterine cancers, among other health benefits.

3. Regular Exercise Enhances Your State of Mind

A study published in *Psychoneuroendocrinology* by Boecker et al., 2008 found that physical activity indeed increases endorphin levels, particularly in the brain, leading to improved mood and a reduction in depressive symptoms.

This research suggests that endorphins and other neurochemicals (like dopamine and serotonin) are released early in a workout, often within the first 10-15 minutes, contributing to the mood-enhancing effects commonly known as a "runner's high." Endorphins, often referred to as "feel-good" hormones help to combat depression and enhance overall mood.

4. Purposeful Exercise Enhances Your Relationships

When you are in great shape and physically fit, you often experience increased energy levels and a noticeable improvement in your overall mood. You will find that you are able to push beyond your previous limits and accomplish more than you thought possible. These positive changes in your physical state can have both direct and indirect effects on your relationships. Enhanced mood, increased confidence and higher energy levels can lead to more fulfilling interactions with others and a greater capacity to engage in meaningful activities.

5. Body-building workouts give you more energy

Regular exercise can indeed boost your energy levels, which in turn can enhance productivity at home and work. Additionally, having fitness goals can provide a sense of purpose and direction. This focus helps increase persistence and keeps you on track as you work towards your objectives. By integrating exercise into your routine, you not only improve your physical health but also strengthen your commitment to personal and professional goals.

6. Keeping Fit Boosts Your Self-Esteem

Regular exercise can indeed have a positive impact on self-esteem and body image, making you feel more confident and comfortable in your appearance. It also fosters social interaction, helping to build connections and reduce feelings of isolation. Additionally, the increased physical fitness and improved mood from exercise can enhance libido and intimacy, contributing to a more fulfilling relationship. Overall, integrating regular physical activity into your life supports not only your physical health but also your emotional and relational well-being.

7. Bodybuilding Improves Your Thinking

The Kingdom of God is said to be within you, connected to your glands. You are a spirit, with a soul, living inside a body. Real life extends beyond what we see, feel, hear, smell, and taste. Exercise helps you clear the mind and change the thought process, improving mind-body coordination and supporting a healthier, more balanced life.

The Kingdom expands as you get closer to reality. As you yield to the Word of God, the Kingdom begins to expand both within and around you. It starts from your spirit and extends to your realm of the soul. This process drives out anything in your soul that does not align with your highest values, through the power of the kingdom within you. As your spirit connects with your mind and emotions, thinking and feeling are greatly improved—you literally become a new creation.

8. Exercises Will Lead to Greater Quality of Life

The impact of physical activity goes beyond weight control. It contributes to a longer life, as evidenced by longevity statistics and life-expectancy data. Regular physical activity also enhances the overall quality of life. Few lifestyle choices have a significant impact on health as engaging in regular exercise.

9. Exercise Relieves Financial Burden

In addition to its profound impact on health, obesity imposes a significant financial burden. The importance of physical activity is increasingly recognized within the public health community. Even moderate physical activity can greatly benefit health and reduce the financial costs associated with managing obesity.

10. Working Out Every Day Will Lower the Risk of Disease

Daily exercise significantly lowers the risk of chronic diseases such as cardiovascular diseases, type 2 diabetes, and some cancers. By improving blood circulation, exercise strengthens the heart, reduces blood pressure, and prevents cholesterol buildup in arteries. Additionally, regular physical activity improves insulin sensitivity, helping to regulate blood sugar and decrease diabetes risk, while supporting weight management to reduce obesity-related health issues.

Exercise also boosts immune function, making the body more resilient to infections and diseases. Moderate daily activity increases immune cell production, enhancing the body's defense against illness.

The World Health Organization (WHO) and the American Heart Association (AHA) recommend at least 150 minutes of moderate-intensity or 75 minutes of vigorous-intensity aerobic activity per week to maintain optimal health.

Ways to Exercise

There are various ways to exercise your mind and body; all you need to do is choose a few that you enjoy. By incorporating a small amount of exercise into your daily routine, you'll feel better than ever, and your body will thank you.

Experts often categorize exercise and physical activity into four types: endurance, strength, balance and flexibility. Engaging in a mix of these activities not only provides more comprehensive benefits but also helps reduce boredom and minimize the risk of injury.

Some activities fit into more than one category. For example, many endurance exercises also build strength, while strength training can help improve balance. Incorporating a variety of activities ensures you get a well-rounded workout that benefits multiple aspects of your fitness.

- **Endurance or aerobic activities** increase your breathing and heart rate, making daily activities easier to perform. Activities such as dancing, jogging, walking, and outdoor work enhance the health of your heart, lungs, and circulatory system, improving overall fitness.

- **Strength exercises** build muscle strength, which is essential for maintaining independence and performing everyday tasks such as climbing stairs and carrying groceries. Examples of strength exercises include lifting weights, using resistance bands and performing bodyweight exercises.

- **Balance exercises** help prevent falls. By improving stability, many lower-body strength exercises also enhance balance. Activities such as standing on one foot and performing heel-to-toe walks are effective for this purpose.

- **Flexibility exercises** stretch your muscles and enhance your range of motion. Improved flexibility provides greater freedom of movement for both exercise and daily activities. Stretches for the shoulders, upper arms and calves are particularly beneficial for achieving this.

Chapter 4

Your Words and Wellness

"Death and life are in the power of the tongue: and they that love it shall eat the fruit thereof." – Proverbs 18:21

In this book, I will reference two levels of words: God's Word and spoken words. Before delving into these concepts, I encourage you to remember that the Word of God, which represents the highest level of communication from God to humanity and is affirmed by our confession, is real.

Words are mighty and creative by nature. God created this world with words, and since we are born of Him and share His attributes, the words we speak have the power to create, shape, and influence our lives and destinies. It concerns me when I encounter believers speaking words of death rather than of life. Such words are unbecoming and do not align with the life-affirming power God intends for us.

The Bible explicitly describes the Word of God as "medicine." God is clear in His will for His children to be well and healthy. Our God, our Heavenly Father, has a purpose for each of us, and to fulfill it, we must be spiritually, mentally, emotionally, and physically whole. We are called to walk in divine wholeness and sound, equipped with a sound mind to grasp the wisdom, knowledge, and understanding He provides.

Recognizing the reality and potency of words is crucial. Your healing begins with your mouth—the faculty of your speech. There is nothing more powerful than speaking God's Word back to Him and applying it to every situation and circumstance you encounter. It is essential to monitor your words carefully. Speak only what God has declared about you in His Word. "For with the heart, man believes unto righteousness, and with the mouth, confession is made unto salvation" (unto health, unto healing, unto wholeness, unto deliverance, and unto victory in your health) (Romans 10:10).

Abraham prayed to God, and God healed Abimelech, his wife, and his female slaves so they could have children again (Genesis 20:17, NIV). The scripture is unequivocal: God healed Abimelech through Abraham's intercession. His wife and maids were also healed so they could be fruitful.

Thus, from the above reference, there is no doubt that prayer and intercession can open the door to healing. The spoken words in prayer have the capacity to heal and restore.

Charles Capps said, "Speak to Your Immune System; It's Listening!"

You should always declare to your Immune system and say, *listen to me: you are filled with the wisdom of God. You discern good from evil, right from wrong. You resist the destroyer and embrace the good. You neither overreact nor underreact, but effectively neutralize every pathogen and abnormal cell. All the microorganisms in my body are balanced and healthy, residing in the exact locations necessary for optimal health. Life prevails in every cell of my body; there is no death. The same spirit that raised Christ from the dead quickens and makes alive every cell in my body. I live out the full span of my life in health and fulfill all that God has for me.*

Let me quickly state this fact: To experience the efficacy of the Word of God, you need to be consistent and diligent in consuming the Word, just as you eat food. Furthermore, the Word must be taken with understanding, much like patients take their medications. Often, as nurses, we crush pills for patients who cannot ingest them due to certain conditions. This is analogous to how we sometimes need to break down the Word of God—His medicine—into more understandable forms, such as different translations.

Obedience: The Key to Preservation from Diseases

"And said, If thou wilt diligently hearken to the voice of the Lord thy God, and wilt do that which is right in His sight, and wilt give ear to His commandments, and keep all His statutes, I will put none of these diseases upon thee, which I have brought upon the Egyptians: for I am the Lord that healeth thee."
— Exodus 15:26 (KJV)

"And He said, If thou wilt diligently hearken to the voice of Jehovah thy God..."
— Exodus 15:26 (ASV)

This scripture is fascinating. I have heeded the voice of the Lord my God and have done what is right in His sight. As a result, He will put none of these diseases upon me. He sent His Word to heal and deliver me from all sickness and disease.

If you want to also enjoy God's preservation from any form of diseases and sicknesses, you must be willing to obey His instructions as revealed in His Word. God would make an edge around you and not allow any of the diseases plaguing the world to come near your dwelling.

The Limitation of Healthcare Systems and Professionals
As a nurse with over thirty years of experience in the healthcare arena, I am continually amazed at how much authority we, as healthcare professionals, sometimes believe we possess—the right to assess and conclude a patient's case. But we are often wrong because we don't possess such a power.

In fact, when you examine the current state of the healthcare system, it is evident that it is deeply flawed and increasingly inadequate. Humanity seems to lack a solution. The impacts of healthcare systems and professionals are noteworthy but it is still evident that we are limited. There is only so little our wisdom and intelligence can do in the myriads of problems that plague the healthcare sector. There are still many unanswered questions and discoveries yet to be made.

However, I want to assure you that the answer lies in the Word of God. That is why I consider myself a messenger and an advocate of God's Word. I want to convey that God's medicine, His Word, can work for anyone who believes and offers hope beyond what conventional medicine provides. God's Word is superior to natural medicine because it cannot be overdosed, works more effectively than a standard dose, has no side effects, and the best news is that it is entirely free.

It is important to note that just as you would adhere to a medical prescription, God's Word must be taken multiple times daily and consistently. It won't be effective if it remains on a shelf. If you don't open your Bible and engage with it, none of the healing verses within will benefit you. Moreover, God's guidance for using His medicine should be followed as diligently and regularly as you would a doctor's prescription—or even more so.

Here is God's direction on His medicine bottle as revealed in Proverbs 4:20–23:

1. "My son, give attention to my words" (verse 20a).

2. "Incline your ear to my sayings" (verse 20b).

3. "Do not let them depart from your eyes" (verse 21a).

4. "Keep them in the midst of your heart" (verse 21b).

When you adhere strictly to that prescription, God's words will become life to you who has found them and radiant health to all your flesh (verse 22). Then it says, "Keep your heart with all diligence, for out of it spring the issues of life" (verse 23). You see, you have a part in keeping this promise to you. That is your responsibility.

In verse 22, the Hebrew word "HEALTH" is translated as "MEDICINE" in many translations of the Bible. Don't forget that for God's medicine to penetrate our bodies and reach the core of our system, we need to consume it with the same seriousness and precision as we would a medical prescription. The only way to do this is by following the prescription God gave us from His Word in Proverbs 4:20–22, as enumerated above.

I have heard this repeatedly from many spiritual health experts: "If you want to walk in divine health, you must saturate yourself with God's Word regarding healing and divine health." I heard someone say, "We cannot get our healing by consistently watching ungodly television shows, nor by watching the negative and discouraging news every day, continually feeding our ear gate and mind gate with the negative things of this world." Your ear and eye are gates to your mind and can adversely affect your life because what gets to your mind can get to your life.

When trusting God for your healing, you must create an atmosphere where the Holy Spirit can operate without hindrance. This allows His love and Blood to saturate and penetrate your very being, enabling healing to flow from the top of your head to the soles of your feet. Having worked in a hospital for over thirty wonderful years, I have seen and treated countless patients with various diseases, such as heart disease, bone disease, head trauma, gallbladder issues, and stomach ailments. There are many chiefs—a term we use in the emergency setting—but ultimately, the doctors make the final diagnosis. It is heartbreaking to see people come into the hospitals and die from diseases. My mother passed away a few years ago from an unknown cause and despite my many years of experience as a nurse, I could not save her, even though I was there at her bedside. There is a better way to live. The Scripture says, "My people perish because of lack of knowledge." (Hosea 4:6) In the scientific world, there are incurable diseases. But with God, by applying His Heavenly medication, there is no disease that cannot be cured. I am convinced that if you have the faith to believe in taking God's Word consistently, as you take your natural pills, there would be no sickness or disease hurting you. God wants you to walk in radiant health. If you constantly experience poor health, then take God's Word daily (even more) and speak it with positive faith over your body until your health springs forth.

I remind nurses to be careful about what we declare and speak over our patients. Negative words should not be used on patients because our words can become a blessing or a curse, bringing healing or sickness, life or death. A consistent affirmation of God's Word over our lives will strengthen every part of our body and make us whole if we are sick. Therefore, it is essential to speak God's words of health and healing over your life if you want to live a healthy and victorious life.

I have also learned over the years that repetition brings forth reality and a good outcome because repetition is the law of deep and lasting impressions. It is not enough to say the Word occasionally and then give up; it should be spoken often and repeatedly from the central core of our being. Therefore, when God's Word is spoken repeatedly over your body, the result is inevitable. Moreover, God wants you to say the word and live the word. That means practicing the word until it becomes automatic and natural. In this way, your faith comes by hearing, so you will not have to struggle over your healing. A songwriter said, "Come, taste and see that the Lord is good." My experience is, "Come, taste and see that the Word is good, and you will find radiant health for your soul and body."

Proverbs 17:22 (NKJV) says, "A merry heart does good, like medicine, but a broken spirit dries the bones." I love this scripture because it speaks volumes about the reality of health and wholeness. As a Registered Nurse for thirty-one years, I have seen many patients return to the hospital because they didn't take their medicine. This principle also applies to receiving divine healing. If you don't take your medicine—God's Word—you might find yourself returning to the hospital with sickness and weakness.

Please don't forget this: Though I am not advocating that drugs and treatments are the ultimate solution, if you do not have faith in your healing and wholeness by the Word of God (His medicine), you must take the doctor's prescription. It will do you good, as God's Word says: "A merry heart doeth good like a medicine" (Proverbs 17:22a, KJV). That tells us that even medicine has a place in our wholeness.

Please pray this prayer now for the Word of God to work in you:

Thank you, Lord, because Your Word is working mightily in me. Now, I am made whole spiritually, physically, emotionally, and relationally, in Jesus' name. Amen.

Chapter 5

Resist Unforgiveness and Anger

"Forgive Fast, Forgive Quickly." — Eva M. Francis

Unforgiveness and anger can have detrimental effects on our physical and mental health. Holding onto grudges and harboring feelings of resentment can lead to increased stress, anxiety, and even depression. Studies have shown that chronic anger and unforgiveness can contribute to a weakened immune system. As well as contributing to higher blood pressure and an increased risk of heart disease. The release of stress hormones in response to anger and unforgiveness can also negatively impact our digestive system, leading to issues such as irritable bowel syndrome and stomach ulcers. Furthermore, the constant state of emotional distress caused by holding onto anger can disrupt sleep patterns and contribute to insomnia.

Overall, the toxic emotions of unforgiveness and anger can manifest in various physical ailments and have long-term consequences on our overall well-being. It is important to address these emotions through forgiveness and healthy coping mechanisms to protect our health and promote healing.

"But I say to you that everyone who is angry with his brother will be liable to judgment; whoever insults his brother will be liable to the council, and whoever says, 'You fool,' will be liable to the hell of fire. So, if you are offering your gift at the altar and there remember that your brother has something against you, leave your gift before the altar and go. First, be reconciled to your brother, and then come and offer your gift."
— Matthew 5:23

I cannot emphasize enough how important it is for you to forgive quickly and walk free of unforgiveness and offense. In the Bible, Esau had all the excuses in the world to hold a grudge against his brother Jacob, who had greatly offended him by taking his father's blessing. Esau could neither forgive nor love his brother. In Genesis 27:4, we are told how Esau harbored unforgiveness and vowed to slay his brother after their father's death. Thank God, according to the scriptures, their mother, Rebecca, intervened. This is a great story to read on the topic of unforgiveness.

How many of us today are so filled with hatred because we choose not to forgive our brothers and sisters? When we allow unforgiveness to settle in our hearts, it does not only affect us spiritually but can also manifest physically in the form of sickness and disease. Holding grudges means we are living out of alignment with our natural default, which is love. God is love, and we were created to love.

A few years ago, I experienced significant hurt due to someone's dishonesty and lack of credibility. I'll spare you the details for now, as that's a topic for another book. To make a long story short, I was consumed by anger and bitterness toward this individual. This anger, along with resentment and bitterness, welled up inside of me until I had to choose between holding onto it or releasing this person through the power of forgiveness. When I chose to forgive and let it go, I felt like a brand-new person. I felt refreshed, renewed, and overwhelmed with the love of God.

The Bible says, "Let all bitterness, wrath, anger, clamor, and evil speaking be put away from you, with all malice" (Ephesians 4:31, NKJV). I truly believe that the Holy Spirit is grieved when we harbor and seal bitterness in our hearts. Many scriptures clearly address refraining from anger, resentment, and bitterness. What this tells you is that God despises these feelings. Until you let go of them, you cannot move forward in God and with God. You will not experience the greatness and the goodness of Your heavenly Father, God. You must address resentment and unforgiveness before they hinder your progress.

I also had another experience where I felt hurt by two individuals who were very close and dear to me in my career. I trusted these two colleagues immensely. They were individuals with whom I laughed, spent lots of time, shared ideas, learned, networked, and so on. After working together for many years, their actions displayed bitterness and resentment when I decided to reinvent my career. What they did caused me significant hurt and pain, leading to deep resentment within me. I thought I had forgiven them because I prayed and entrusted the situation to the Lord. However, whenever their names were mentioned, I would feel a burning sensation in my stomach. It became clear that, despite verbally claiming forgiveness, I had not truly forgiven them. This unresolved pain affected me physically, and I ended up in the emergency room with ongoing abdominal pain. All the tests conducted showed that I was medically sound.

Then, one morning while praying, the Lord revealed to me that I had not truly forgiven those who had hurt me, and this was causing my abdominal pain. I argued with the Lord, insisting, "Yes, Lord, I know that I have forgiven them."

Suddenly, I realized that it was the Lord who had placed it in my heart that I hadn't truly forgiven them. The Lord said, "If you have forgiven them, you would not feel the way you are currently feeling. You think about them with so much hurt, anger, and bitterness." He continued, "When you begin to think about them without any bitterness, then you know that you have forgiven. When you begin to think about them with thoughts of love and kindness, then you will know that you have truly forgiven them."

"Forgiveness is evident when you begin to walk in the love of God for these individuals," says God. Forgiveness is evident when you start to experience peace. Immediately, my eyes were opened. God showed me that I needed to forgive them and forgive myself for

24

anything I had done that might have triggered their behavior. Often, we are quick to blame others and delay forgiveness without considering what role we may have played in the situation. Let us not be so quick to blame others. Instead, reflect on what you might have done to trigger these circumstances. God also reminded me to start praying for their families, their health, their careers, businesses, and their success—and to act as if they had never wronged me. I should focus on praying for their welfare for the next few days, rather than dwelling on my situation. I obeyed, believing that this would help me feel better and receive all the blessings the Lord has provided me. Don't miss out on what God has planned for your life—start walking in love, grace, peace, and forgiveness.

The Lord also showed me Romans 9:33 from the New American Standard Bible: "Behold, I lay in Zion a stone of stumbling and a rock of offense, and he who believes in Him will not be disappointed."

When I took the step to obey the Lord, I felt better. The pain and bad feelings began to go away. Then, on that day, I said to myself, "I will not hold on to any more grudges or unforgiveness." At that moment, I experienced a supernatural deliverance from physical pain and nausea. I felt well immediately, so I sent one of the individuals an email and later called the other. The outcome was complete and instant deliverance. No, it was not easy; it took me a while to get to that level.

I also have a friend who was a mentee for some time. One day, she confided in me that she was doing everything she knew was right but could not get a job. She applied everywhere, and although God promised her that He had a job lined up for her, she had not seen any success in that area. During the conversation, she revealed to me that there were many individuals in her life whom she thought about with sadness in her heart because of what "they did" to her. Again, we love to say what others have done, but God also wants us to take responsibility for our actions and behaviors, as well as set others free from bondage through the power of forgiveness. After she spent time in prayer and forgave her offenders, she got her dream job, and at the time of writing this book, she has been enjoying massive success.

I cannot overemphasize how important it is to let go of the poison and toxicity of unforgiveness. It is debilitating, terrible for your health, and poisonous to your spirit. It is an infection that can spread into your inner being. Start working on letting go of bitterness and unforgiveness today. Let it go and ask God for His love and forgiveness in your heart. Many people ruin their health and their lives while preventing the blessings and favor of God by merely holding on to past hurt and pain. Sadly, this is also very prevalent among believers.

If you continue to drink the toxin and poison of unforgiveness, it will only lead to an adverse outcome, and the only one who will be affected by this action is you. It is bondage and torture to have hurtful thoughts playing inside your head. You may want to take revenge; you may even want negative things to happen to those people who hurt you. But I come to declare to you, by the Blood of Jesus Christ and by the unction of God's Word, if that's you, let it go, and you'll be glad you did.

You will be relieved of all bitterness and the sins that easily beset you. Your prayers will be answered, and even if the other individual does not receive your forgiveness, you have done your part, and you will be set free. Nothing tastes as good as freedom does.

God wants His children to live free; whom the Son sets free is free indeed. We can be free from condemnation and free from judgment. Hallelujah! When we forgive, we allow God to work freely in us. Many walk around sick and in pain, unable to receive healing despite the many hands that have been laid on them, the changes made in their eating habits, or the higher doses of medications taken.

The answer is in forgiveness and in letting go of the hurt and pain. Speak positive words over the situation, walk in humility, and watch God work in your life. Now, is this going to be easy to do? The answer is no, not at all. It is not something you can do on your own. You will need to ask the Holy Spirit to step in and help you. The Holy Spirit is our Helper.

I'll reiterate: He is your Helper.

As you read these words, my desire is for you to experience the power of forgiveness made possible by our Lord and Savior, Jesus Christ.

Forgiveness is never the easiest thing to do, but let me say this: "It is a very necessary element to live the healthy life that God calls us to live." I remember reading an article some time ago from John Hopkins Medicine titled *Forgiveness: Your Health Depends on It*. It says that studies have found the act of forgiveness can reap huge rewards for one's health, lowering the risk of heart disease, improving cholesterol levels, improving sleep, reducing pain, normalizing blood pressure, and decreasing levels of anxiety and stress. Studies have also found that many individuals are naturally more forgiving, while others hold grudges for a very long time. Consequently, those who are more forgiving tend to live more satisfying lives with less anxiety, depression, and hostility. Have you ever wondered what this world would be like if we were all more forgiving of each other?

Another factual key that not everyone will agree on is when you choose to release an offense. Others may say to you, "You are silly. After all they did to you, you will just let it go like that?" But don't listen to those voices; remember that there is power in being obedient to God.

Another essential fact about resentment and unforgiveness is that it causes stress. It is well documented in many research studies that stress is a major cause of many diseases in the body. The number one cause and risk factor for deadly diseases is stress-related. I cannot begin to tell you how many individuals I have seen admitted to the hospital over the years because of high-level stress, which is often masked with medications.

So, how do you start relieving yourself of stress? You can start by relaxing, taking deep breaths, and meditating upon the Word of God. Nothing heals faster than addressing the cause. If you can identify the cause, take care of it first before things get complicated health-wise. Every day, you must make every effort to renew your mind with God's Word. That's another remedy for health and wellness. Everything starts with the mind. It is when we begin to have healthy thoughts that our words will produce fruit. So, the lesson about forgiveness is this:

No matter how healthy you think you are by eating well, taking supplements, exercising, drinking alkaline water, and eating vegetables. As well as getting adequate rest, relaxing, juicing every day, or eating a vegan meal - harboring unforgiveness, bitterness, sadness, resentment, fear, jealousy, anxiety, or depression in your heart, you are not truly healthy. Health and wholeness start from within.

Prayer:

Lord, help me to forgive anyone who has hurt me in the past. You have said in Your Word that if we do not forgive, our prayers will be hindered. And because I want You to hear my prayer so that I can stay healthy, I forgive myself and my enemies. Today, I choose to walk in divine forgiveness. Amen.

Thank You that my health and youth are renewed like that of an eagle because of Your forgiving power.

Chapter 6

Hydration- Drinking From the Fountain of Living Water

"With joy you will draw water from the wells of salvation."

— (Isaiah 12:3, NIV)

Water is often referred to as the *"water of life"* in the Bible, symbolizing purification, renewal, and sustenance. The significance of hydration in maintaining health and wellness is echoed in biblical teachings, which emphasize the importance of caring for our bodies as temples of the Holy Spirit. In this chapter, we will explore the scientific implications of hydration on our physical and mental well-being, alongside the biblical wisdom that underscores the importance of proper hydration.

The Science of Hydration

Our bodies are fearfully and wonderfully made, intricately designed to function optimally when properly hydrated. As mentioned in the Bible, in Psalm 139:14: "I praise you because I am fearfully and wonderfully made; your works are wonderful, I know that full well." Water is essential for regulating body temperature, facilitating nutrient absorption, and eliminating waste from the body. Neglecting proper hydration can disrupt these vital processes and lead to a myriad of health issues.

Dehydration, both physical and spiritual, can have profound effects on our well-being. Just as our bodies require water to function, our spirits require the living water of God's Word for nourishment and sustenance. Jesus declared in John 4:14, "But whoever drinks the water I give them will never thirst. Indeed, the water I give them will become in them a spring of water welling up to eternal life." Just as physical dehydration can lead to fatigue and weakness, spiritual dehydration can leave us feeling spiritually drained and disconnected from God.

The Impact of Hydration on Physical Performance
Proper hydration is essential for honoring our bodies as temples of the Holy Spirit and maximizing our physical potential. The apostle Paul reminds us in 1 Corinthians 6:19-20: "Do you not know that your bodies are temples of the Holy Spirit, who is in you, whom you have received from God? You are not your own; you were bought at a price. Therefore, honor God with your bodies." Staying hydrated enables us to care for our bodies and fulfill the purpose for which God has created us.

Athletes and individuals engaged in physical activity can draw inspiration from the biblical analogy of running the race of faith with endurance (Hebrews 12:1). Just as athletes must fuel their bodies with water to perform at their best, believers must nourish their spirits with the living water of God's Word to run the race of faith with perseverance and endurance.

Hydration and Spiritual Well-being
In addition to its physical benefits, hydration also plays a significant role in our spiritual well-being. The psalmist declares in Psalm 42:1: "As the deer pants for streams of water, so my soul pants for you, my God." Just as physical dehydration can lead to thirst, our souls long for the living water of God's presence and Word to quench our spiritual thirst.

Staying hydrated spiritually involves cultivating a daily practice of prayer, meditation, and reflection on Scripture. Just as we replenish our bodies with water throughout the day, we must continually refresh our spirits with the life-giving water of God's Word to nourish our souls and maintain spiritual vitality.

What fountain are you drinking from?

Jeremiah 2:13 (NKJV) says, "For My people have committed two evils: They have forsaken Me, the fountain of living waters, and hewn themselves cisterns—broken cisterns that can hold no water."

This portion of Scripture speaks profoundly about where and how we get filled in life. Are we going to the fountain of living waters to be forever filled, satisfied, and made clean (John 4:14; Hebrews 10:22; Revelation 22:1)? Or are we going to our dirty sewage water wells that hold nothing but murky, disgusting, and unclean water? These latter things in the world that promise to fill us up but never do.

In the scripture above, we see that these people (much like us) have forsaken the Lord—the fountain of living waters—and instead pursued fleeting pleasures and satisfaction when all we need is found in our Lord and Savior Jesus Christ.

This verse parallels what Jesus said in John 7:38, when He stood up and cried, "If you believe in Me, out of your belly will flow rivers of living water." The Holy Spirit fills our wells until they overflow, so that we are always satisfied in Him when we come to drink.

Are you an exclusive drinker? Are you finding pleasure and fulfillment in Christ alone? Or are you turning to things in the world—to other people—and trying to fill up from them? This is a call for self-examination. Christ specifically wants you to seek His grace continuously. He wants you to know Him and to make Him known. He wants you to drink from His well of living water alone and not any other success.

Have you ever strayed away from Christ for various reasons? How did you feel during that period of straying? I believe it was a frustrating and unfulfilling time for you.

A few years ago, I was always so busy. Then I asked myself, amid all the 'busyness'—how did I get so busy? I couldn't really understand why I had so many things going on at the same time. When our lives are so busy and cluttered, it can be challenging to stay focused and hear what God the Father is saying to us. At such times, it becomes very hard for us to give thanks and praise to God, and we miss out on what He is saying to us. I must confess that I have missed God many times in my walk, and the main reason was simply that I found myself overly busy. If you are too busy to take care of yourself, what you are saying to God is that you are too busy to enjoy Him. Lots of times, we are unnecessarily busy. We can do without some of the things we do at times. I have learned over the years to ascertain my priorities. Are our priorities always in order? No! But if any Christian wants to live a victorious life, they must make the conscious decision to spend time and get acquainted with the Lord Jesus Christ. Let us make a quality decision today to live and enjoy all the things that God has provided for us without being too busy.

Natural Water

If you are a nurse, a physician, or any other healthcare worker reading this book, you will attest to the fact that if a sick patient is brought through the doors of any hospital, the first thing a nurse or a doctor will think about (as far as treatment is concerned) is assessing the fluid status of the patient. In a situation of cardiac arrest, the first thing we think of is administering a large volume of fluids. During the hospital stay, when a patient is not receiving any form of parenteral (intravenous) fluids, there is an immediate assumption that this patient is almost ready or ready to be discharged. I am saying this to reinforce the importance of hydration.

I once read a book by Dr. Batmanghelidj, MD, *Your Body's Many Cries for Water*. After reading this book, my perception of water changed. The book explains that a lack of water in the body—chronic dehydration—is the root cause of many painful degenerative

32

diseases. I received a strong revelation based on research that water is the answer to most health crises and that if we drink more water, we will live a victorious and healthy life.

Another good book I have read on the subject of water is by Pastor Stanley Moore, Sr. of Words of Life Fellowship Church in North Miami Beach. Pastor Stan provides a spiritual perspective on the health benefits of drinking water. One day, I was in church, and I received a revelation from the Lord through Pastor Stanley's teaching. He mentioned in the book that water would add years to your life and life to your years. Below is what I have in my notes from Pastor Stan, and with his permission to do so, I will quote him:

God has provided many different means and avenues whereby healing and health can be obtained. One of the simplest, inexpensive, and readily accessible ways is through hydration. Drinking water can positively affect your spirit, soul, and body, and it will revolutionize your life. Through this simple God-given resource of water, one can enjoy more mental and emotional health and well-being and live a victorious life full of energy, vigor, vitality, and the joy of the Lord. You will not only be adding years to your life, but you will also be adding life to your years as you learn how to live well with water.

Take note of that, please.

I know of a lady who received her healing and whose health has since improved because God told her to drink more water. She was suffering from chronic belly pain when, one day, she received a revelation from God to increase her water intake. After a few days, she was healed, and that sickness and disease never came back again. She said that instead of thinking about food all the time, as she would typically do, she now thinks about water. That bears witness to my spirit, and I am trying to do the same as well. It is good for my health, and it shouldn't take much to convince anyone of the same. All you need to do is try it.

Furthermore, water is vital to our living and well-being. The need for it can hardly be overstated. As humans, we are composed of approximately 70 percent water, and nearly every aspect of our body's function requires fluid and proper hydration. If you studied science in school, you might recall that early science classes taught us about the benefits of water. It constitutes much of the medium that helps our cells communicate with each other. It is a fact that humans can survive only a few days without water—fewer than they can without food.

You might ask: Is eight glasses of water a day necessary? Well, the answer depends on many factors. The first thing to consider would be the person's general health status. Some people can tolerate that much, while others cannot, depending on their health conditions. Individuals with chronic pain need to evaluate their water intake to ensure they are drinking enough. Water is a source of life. Clinically, patients have noticed improvements in treatments they were already pursuing—such as chiropractic work, acupuncture, or massage—just by being better hydrated.

I have had personal experience with proper hydration, and it relieved me of my pain. Some people claim they can do without drinking water, but that is hard for me to fathom. At times, I even hear people say, "I don't drink water" or "I don't like water." It bothers me to hear such statements. As a healthcare provider, my goal is to help others understand what water can do for and within our bodies.

The questions I ask about drinking water are: Is the person engaged in activities that increase water loss (such as sweating)? Is the person working out extensively? Or do they have a job that frequently puts them outside in the heat? Does the person drink a lot of coffee or soft drinks (sodas)? Coffee can act as a diuretic, which means it may increase urination. A lot of coffee, in this case, would be defined as three or more cups a day. Regular or diet soft drinks pose many health issues. People who drink multiple cans of soda a day may not be getting enough water.

One of the most significant problems people face by drinking high volumes of coffee or soft drinks is that their "addiction" to these beverages eventually replaces water and becomes their primary form of hydration. Again, coffee is a diuretic, so an excessive amount of it can worsen the water balance in the body. Conversely, high coffee intake could cause losses of minerals and calcium. You need to understand that hydration cannot come from any other source but water—water is absolutely irreplaceable. I have nothing against coffee, but this is a fact.

There is very little data on exactly how much water a person should drink. However, the old suggestion of eight-ounce glasses a day may still be a realistic guideline. Athletes in training should target eighty to ninety ounces or more, depending on their level of perspiration. If the urine appears dark yellow, then water intake needs to be increased. Typically, the color of urine should be pale yellow. One study documented that even experienced long-distance runners did not always gauge how dehydrated they were. Another fact is that people receiving bodywork therapies like massage or chiropractic treatments should also be drinking high amounts of water to best utilize those therapies. I would suggest that coffee drinkers limit their daily intake to one or two cups while meeting their water goals for the day.

Another question we should examine is this: What type of water is best? These days, there is bottled water, flavored water, vitamin water, and, of course, tap water. The best source for drinking and cooking is water filtered through a reverse osmosis system. This is a very high-grade filter that can be installed under your kitchen sink by a local water company. However, any other form of regular water— whether tap or bottled—is still better than soda.

Vitamins and specialty waters can become problematic due to added sugars. Some promise extra vitamins when, in fact, they contain very few. The truth is that water doesn't need to provide anything other than water—it is efficient enough. While bottled water popularized hydration, its boom also triggered a huge influx of plastic bottles being dumped into our environment, which allows certain chemicals like phthalates to leach into the groundwater and then into our bodies. These pose various risks, including cancer. The best thing to do is to transport water in stainless steel or glass bottles. And if you have plastic bottles, don't allow them to sit in the sun.

Moreover, don't use plastics to carry or heat water, as this might increase chemical leaching. Use a glass or a pitcher, and be sure to drink the natural gift of water. Clean, pure, and fresh water will rejuvenate and revitalize you, helping your body get back into balance.

Why is the Bible and Water of Significance to Christians?
The Bible and water are deeply connected. Water is mentioned 722 times in Scripture. That is less than God, Jesus, heaven, or love, but many more times than faith, hope, prayer, or even worship. When I found that out, I found it very interesting and wanted to learn more about the significance of water in the Bible.

The first time water is mentioned in Scripture is in Genesis 1:2 (NLT):
"The earth was formless and empty, and darkness covered the deep waters. And the Spirit of God was hovering over the surface of the waters."

Before there was anything—light, sun, moon, earth, plants, or living creatures—there was water. He continues to bathe His creation in water as a sign of His care. The last and final time water is mentioned is in Revelation 22:17 (NLT):

The Spirit and the bride say, 'Come.' Let anyone who hears this say, 'Come.' Let anyone who is thirsty come. Let anyone who desires drink freely from the water of life."

Throughout the Bible, water is frequently referenced. Many passages link water to God's creative, blessing, and saving work. This highlights the significance of water in our spiritual lives. These are just a few examples of both the literal and figurative uses of water in Scripture.

With over seven hundred references to water in the Bible, I believe that God has something to say to us. I urge you to read, study, and meditate on this further. The Bible and water are crucial for any believer. I would say that these are two of the main means by which God's power and grace are revealed to us—but only if we seek them out and accept His gift.

The Bible and water sustain both our physical and spiritual lives. They remind us of our Creator and Savior, who unites us with the Spirit, transforms, and purifies both the world and every believer. As believers, if we continue to take the Bible as well as water for granted, we may have difficulties in our physical bodies then, consequently, in our spiritual lives.

When believers in Jesus accept, cherish, respect, and honor both the Bible and water as gifts from God that are freely given to us, we will find our reservoirs of spiritual and physical nourishment.

Isaiah 12:2-3 (NIV) says:

"Surely God is my salvation; I will trust and not be afraid. The Lord, the Lord himself, is my strength and my defense; he has become my salvation. With joy, you will draw water from the wells of salvation."

We will then be able to draw on the Lord and all that our King has for us as His children, with joy, from the wells of salvation. Have you ever heard the saying that the natural mirrors and explains the spiritual? Well, it does, and here is one example of this principle. On day five of creation, we find in Genesis 1:20a (KJV) that God said, "Let the waters bring forth abundantly the moving creature that hath life..." This passage shows us that life emerges from water. Drink an adequate amount of water and begin to experience the physical joys of "better living."

On day five of creation, we find in Genesis 1:20a (KJV) that God said, "Let the waters bring forth abundantly the moving creature that hath life..." This passage shows us that life emerges from the water. This concept is also true in the natural birth process. After conception, we continue to develop and grow in what is essentially a sack of water inside the womb. When a woman is in labor and the baby is about to be born, we wait for her water to break so that the baby can come forth into life.

Also, physical birth (water birth) must come before spiritual birth, as we see in John 3:1-5 (NIV), when Nicodemus, a ruler of the Jews, inquired of Jesus:

"Now there was a Pharisee, a man named Nicodemus, who was a member of the Jewish ruling council. He came to Jesus at night and said, 'Rabbi, we know that you are a teacher who has come from God. For no one could perform the signs you are doing if God were not with him.' Jesus replied, 'Very truly I tell you, no one can see the kingdom of God unless they are born again.' 'How can someone be born when they are old?' Nicodemus asked. 'Surely they cannot enter a second time into their mother's womb to be born!' Jesus answered, 'Very truly I tell you, no one can enter the kingdom of God unless they are born of water and the Spirit.' "

Definition of Water According to God's Word
Water symbolizes God's Word in many places throughout the Bible. In both Psalms and Ephesians, water is a symbol of God's Word:
"That He might sanctify and cleanse her with the washing of water by the word."

In Isaiah 55:10-11 (NIV), water is a simile for the knowledge of God:

"As the rain and the snow come down from heaven and do not return to it without watering the earth and making it bud and flourish, so that it yields seed for the sower and bread for the eater, so is my word that goes out from my mouth: It will not return to me empty but will accomplish what I desire and achieve the purpose for which I sent it."

In Hosea 6:3 (NIV), the rains are a sign of the presence of God:

"Let us acknowledge the LORD; let us press on to acknowledge him. As surely as the sun rises, he will appear; he will come to us like the winter rains, like the spring rains that water the earth."

Finally, in Amos 5:24 (NIV), water represents social justice:

"But let justice roll on like a river, righteousness like a never-failing stream!"

Believers in Christ Jesus would do well to read, study, and meditate on the Word of God. Engaging with the Bible can have a cleansing effect on us, much like water cleanses and refreshes. This leads to the next topic in our discussion of the Bible and water.

The Bible and Water Speak of Purification and Cleansing

Water also serves as a means of purification and cleansing. In Exodus, we read that Moses was instructed to make a bronze basin and fill it with water. This serves as another example of how the natural mirrors and explains the spiritual.

Furthermore, in the scripture earlier quoted, "That He might sanctify and cleanse her with the washing of water by the word" (Ephesians 5:26, NKJV), we see that it is a means God uses to cleanse us from all sins and righteousness and make us holy and sanctified for His use.

Chapter 7

God's Word Is the Ultimate

"He sent His word and healed them and delivered

them from their destructions." ~ Psalm 107:20

This is one of my favorite healing scriptures. I have stood by this scripture many times for my healing. A more surefire way to walk in the healing virtue of our dear Lord and Savior, Jesus Christ, is to speak God's words over our bodies, day and night.

A friend of mine, who also attends my church (Words of Life), informed me that she speaks God's healing Word over her body, even though she is well and in no pain, free from sickness and disease. She said that this is how she wards off diseases from attacking her body, and because of that, even though she is in her sixties, she takes no medication. Isn't that a great way to live the abundant life that God has promised us?

As a veteran nurse, I spent most of my career working in hospitals with many great doctors who are highly knowledgeable about the disease process. However, many times, our doctors leave patients with very little hope.

This chapter is meant to inform you that despite the hopelessness you may have heard concerning your condition or situation, God's Word works, and it supersedes what any physician may tell you or has told you. I have seen and prayed with families whose loved ones received a "doom and gloom" report—they are still alive today, enjoying the sweetness and the fullness of a beautiful life God has given them. If you or any of your loved ones have been sick and have gotten a final diagnosis from physicians, I am here to declare to you that God's Word supersedes. No matter what the doctor says or the situation may be, God's Word has the final say. I find strength in, "God's Word is a lamp unto my feet and a light unto my path." (Psalm 119:105)

Despite the genetic, hormonal, and risk factors, as well as the family history that you may hear about—though they have clinical merit—I believe that God's Word has the final authority. That's the reason why I love it so much. I implore you to do the same.

A few years ago, I was working in the intensive care unit of a local hospital. I didn't know as much about the Word of God as I do now. A patient had undergone surgery, and the surgeon delivered terrible news to the family. (I will not go into the details for the sake of confidentiality). The patient's family was told that the patient would not live for more than a few weeks. They responded, "Doctor, we do not believe that." They got together, prayed, and asserted their authority through the Word of God, rebuking the spirit of death and canceling the negative words spoken over their loved ones by the doctors. Many times, we may inadvertently contribute to the negative words we speak over our patients.

Guess what? Their family member ended up walking out of the hospital alive and well. But the doctor had said, "Miracles don't happen so easily." To which I responded, "You bet, miracles do happen, my friend." I could go on and on with so many great stories. That is why I can confidently say that we serve a God who heals, called Jehovah Rapha. He is the Great Physician.

Over the years, I have consistently told my staff that we should allow patients and their family members to believe and pray for the well-being of their loved ones. If they do, it does not matter what we, as caregivers and healthcare workers, say.

If the patient and the family believe that their loved one will be healed, all we need to do as healthcare providers (if we are believers too) is to believe with them and give them the opportunity to see the manifestation. We should not hold them in bondage. Many times, we hold them hostage because we are looking at the situation from a medical standpoint. I believe it is vital to give them that space and, if appropriate, create an atmosphere for healing to take place.

Yes, we have a duty and a responsibility as healthcare workers to do our clinical jobs, but we should not put or throw a spanner in the works that prevents families from taking a spiritual approach. Let them be who they are spiritually.

We should not hold patients hostage because of their beliefs. If families want to sing and pray, we should allow it. I was very glad when The Joint Commission, a healthcare accreditation body, stated that healthcare organizations were being surveyed on being patient-centered. That shows how much priority we give to patients and families. I believe that patients are the most important part of the healthcare equation and that they must be respected, embraced, and empowered to believe in their rights. Patients and families should not be ridiculed because they have a strong spiritual belief, whether you agree with it or not, especially if you do not understand their faith. If they want to pray in tongues (supernatural prayer language), let them pray in tongues—as long as they are not disturbing other patients.

Nurses should allow and promote those holy moments. Our responsibility is to touch their lives as best we can and make a difference every time through every contact. Medical science commands a lot of respect, but it should not draw the line on anyone's life.

I want you to see another thing: evidence abounds on the interconnection between medical science and the Holy Bible. Luke, the author of the Gospel that bears his name, was a medical doctor, as confirmed in Colossians 4:14. I am sure he was a great doctor and evidence-based in his practice. In the Gospel he authored, Luke spoke many times about sicknesses and diagnoses. His Greek origin and practice as a physician explain his scientific and orderly approach to the book and why he gave impressive attention to detail in his account. Luke was also very compassionate toward the poor, the sick, the hurt, and the sinful. In his Gospel, I see where he sets an example for all of us in the healthcare field to follow—to be great caregivers and to be caring and compassionate. We can follow in his footsteps.

Over the years, I've learned that the more patient and compassionate we are as nurses, the faster our patients recover. In other words, our attitude determines their recovery process in the hospital. God has entrusted these patients to our care, and we will give an account of our time with them. I repeat: there is a link between the Bible and medical science. When the Scripture says, "Let fruit be your food and leaves be your medicine" (Ezekiel 47:12), we see a hint of that link.

Nonetheless, everything should be done in moderation, for God is a God of balance. In my opinion, one cannot go wrong by drinking herbal teas. When I first discovered that scripture, I was in awe to see that the Bible gives us a blueprint as to how we should walk, talk, live, and—most of all—how we should eat and drink. Is it any wonder that all nutritionists tell you to eat vegetables or, rather, fruits and leaves, as Scripture says? Hear me now, friends and family; this is scriptural. It is in the Bible, and thus, it supersedes everything.

I remember reading an article where someone said that the Word of God is the only authority. That holds so much truth. If more Christians took God earnestly at His Word, more of us would walk in health and peace (wholeness). Giving God's Word its rightful place in everything will cause us to be instant winners. When we put our faith (to believe and act), our hearts, and our trust in His Word, we will always please God.

Let me tell you a story from the Bible, found in Matthew 8:5-13 (NKJV), about a man who puts God's Word first in his life:

Now when Jesus had entered Capernaum, a centurion came to Him, pleading with Him, saying, 'Lord, my servant is lying at home paralyzed, dreadfully tormented.' "

And Jesus said to him, "I will come and heal him." The centurion answered and said, "Lord, I am not worthy that You should come under my roof. But only speak a word, and my servant will be healed. For I also am a man under authority, having soldiers under me: And I say to this one, 'Go,' and he goes; and to another, 'Come,' and he comes; and to my servant, 'Do this,' and he does it."

When Jesus heard it, He marveled and said to those who followed, "Assuredly, I say to you, I have not found such great faith, not even in Israel! And I say to you that many will come from east and west and sit down with Abraham, Isaac, and Jacob in the kingdom of heaven. But the sons of the kingdom will be cast out into outer darkness. There will be weeping and gnashing of teeth." Then Jesus said to the centurion, "Go your way; and as you have believed, so let it be done for you." And his servant was healed that same hour. "

Did you see that? The centurion gave priority to the Word of God, and as a result, he received the answer to his problem. What would you do in such a situation? Put God's Word first. It supersedes everything else.

Let me show you the importance of meditating on God's Word. Through meditation on the Word of God, we can learn how to quiet our minds and control our thoughts. That brings healing to our mind and body.

If we could understand and catch a glimpse of what God's Word means to us and how we should obey Him, we could spend much less on medical bills in our country. Yes, God's Word supersedes everything—including conditions and the bills. We become what we meditate upon. If we continually ponder on God's Words, health, healing, and wholeness, they will surely come to pass. Health will be our portion. God's Word transforms and heals from within, and that is why meditation is important for healing. By this, I mean meditating on godly things, particularly the Word of God. With it, you set the healing process in motion from the inside out.

I want to declare again that God's Word supersedes what any doctor says—every time. But your faith is what will make it happen for you. Are you a believer today? Or are you just listening to what everyone says, including "Doctor Google"? I implore you to stop taking advice from negative sources, including those that offer divergent views from the Word of God.

Here's a prayer in honor of God's Word:

Heavenly Father, You said in Your Word that we should hide Your Word in our hearts so that we might not sin against You (Psalm 119:11). I believe in Your Word, Lord; now help me to meditate upon it day and night. We become what we meditate upon, and therefore I want to walk in Your healing anointing day and night. Thank You for Your Word, which is life and radiant health to me. Your Word is settled in my heart, and it gives me joy and peace. I also thank You that when man says NO, You, Jesus Christ, say YES. This is my prayer today, in Jesus' name. Amen.

Chapter 8

The Bitter Truth About Sugar

"It is not good to eat too much honey, nor is it honorable to search out matters that are too deep."

- Proverbs 25:27 NIV

More than ever before, sweet treats and sugary substances are greatly loved and consumed. Sugar contents have now become a must-have in most diets—from decadent desserts to sugary beverages. And they surely give us this momentarily pleasure but they don't spare us from the long-term consequences of consuming much sugar.

Americans are so addicted to this deadly substance called sugar. We also justify our cravings at times by saying that we are only eating healthy sugar. Believe me, friends: sugar is sugar. Let me break down the difference for you. Natural sugar differs significantly from refined sugar. This may sometimes confuse the public because, at times, a product might bear a label that says, "No sugar added." To many individuals, this information means there is no sugar. However, that is not the case, so be very careful in reading labels. Natural sugar can be categorized as a single sugar. The body can absorb sugar in its single or mono form.

According to *Harvard Medical School* and *Health Publishing*, "Too much added sugar can be one of the greatest threats to cardiovascular disease." Another study conducted at Harvard concluded that individuals who consume 17% to 21% of their calories from added sugar had a 38% higher risk of dying from cardiovascular disease compared with those who consume 8% of their calories as added sugar.

Basically, the studies revealed that the higher the sugar intake, the greater the risk for heart disease. Understand that if you want to live a long and healthy life, sugar is certainly not your friend.

As children growing up in the rural parts of Jamaica, we enjoyed drinking everything with large amounts of sugar. My childhood memories are filled with moments with my mother (who is now in heaven—God bless her darling heart). She owned a grocery shop in the hills of a place called Mount Pleasant, Macca Tree, St. Catherine. When I went to high school in Spanish Town, I was always afraid to say where I was from because the kids would laugh and tease me about the name of my community. I grew up watching my mother drink sodas almost every day. To her, she was "quenching her thirst." What she did not realize at that time was that the best thirst-quencher is "good, sweet fresh water." I can clearly remember her drinking Kola Champagne soda, especially on Sunday nights, with cornmeal sweet pudding—it was a very tasty snack then, and we all enjoyed it. If you are reading this book and hail from the island of Jamaica, I am sure you catch the reference. I liked it then, and believe me, such old "habits" haven't and won't die off at all—not now, not when I come across them again.

That was my mum's eating habit then... She did not know any better. Then, she developed diabetes, which was very difficult to control due to her lifestyle and eating habits. Back then, we only knew that sugar was sweet and that it tasted good. Nevertheless, the title of this chapter is "The Bitter Truth about Sugar." I could just as well have named it "Sugar: The Sweet, Silent Killer." I read an article entitled "The 126 Reasons Why Sugar Is a Killer," which I will discuss later in this chapter. But first, let us explore what sugar is. The term "sugar" is used to describe a wide range of compounds that vary in sweetness. Common sugars include glucose, fructose, galactose, sucrose, lactose, and maltose. Most of the sugar in the American diet comes from sugars added to food products. It is practically in everything that we eat or drink, and one can become addicted easily.

The body interprets and handles all types of sugars the same way. The resulting simple sugars go directly into the bloodstream. The pancreas then releases a hormone called insulin, which is crucial for removing sugar from the bloodstream and into cells to be used as energy. If the body is not secreting the proper amount of insulin, the sugar will remain unprocessed in the bloodstream and can cause damage to the heart, blood vessels, and kidneys once diabetes develops. There are healthy carbohydrates, including vegetables, brown rice, and sweet potatoes, which are beneficial for the body compared to this substance, which harms our health and wellness. This is not a substance we should entertain in our homes. Consider this: everything we eat or drink contains sugar. Sugar disrupts the body's chemistry and devastates the endocrine and immune systems, contributing to both acute and chronic conditions.

The pervasive presence of sugar in our modern diet has raised concerns about its impact on our health and well-being. While sugar may provide a momentary burst of sweetness and pleasure, the hidden dangers it poses to our bodies are far-reaching and profound. Extensive research and scientific studies have implicated sugar in a myriad of health issues that can adversely affect both our physical and mental well-being.

51 Ways Sugar Can Ruin Your Health:

1. Increases the risk of obesity.
2. Contributes to insulin resistance.
3. Raises blood sugar levels.
4. Promotes inflammation in the body.
5. Leads to fatty liver disease.

6. Raises the risk of type 2 diabetes.
7. Contributes to metabolic syndrome.
8. Increases the risk of heart disease.
9. Promotes the growth of cancer cells.
10. Contributes to non-alcoholic fatty liver disease.
11. Impairs cognitive function and memory.
12. Raises the risk of Alzheimer's disease.
13. Contributes to hormonal imbalances.
14. Increases the risk of gout.
15. Promotes tooth decay and cavities.
16. Contributes to acne and skin issues.
17. Raises the risk of kidney disease.
18. Contributes to mood swings and depression.
19. Increases the risk of anxiety disorders.
20. Promotes oxidative stress in the body.
21. Raises the risk of chronic inflammation.
22. Contributes to autoimmune disorders.
23. Increases the risk of osteoporosis.
24. Promotes cellular aging and wrinkles.
25. Raises the risk of hypertension.
26. Impairs immune function.
27. Contributes to digestive issues such as bloating and gas.
28. Increases the risk of irritable bowel syndrome.
29. Promotes candida overgrowth.
30. Raises the risk of yeast infections.
31. Contributes to chronic fatigue and low energy levels.
32. Impairs sleep quality and disrupts circadian rhythms.
33. Raises the risk of hormone-related cancers.
34. Promotes insulin spikes and crashes.
35. Increases the risk of fatty deposits in arteries.
36. Contributes to joint pain and inflammation.
37. Raises the risk of gallstones.
38. Promotes the development of cataracts.
39. Contributes to muscle cramps and spasms.

40. Increases the risk of metabolic acidosis.

41. Promotes the growth of harmful gut bacteria.

42. Raises the risk of food allergies and sensitivities.

43. Contributes to poor wound healing.

44. Increases the risk of skin conditions such as eczema.

45. Promotes sugar cravings and addictive behavior.

46. Raises the risk of gestational diabetes.

47. Contributes to menstrual irregularities.

48. Increases the risk of erectile dysfunction.

49. Promotes the development of fatty tumors.

50. Raises the risk of liver cirrhosis.

51. Contributes to premature aging and decreased longevity.

These fifty-one ways illustrate the wide-ranging and profound effects that excessive sugar consumption can have on our health and well-being. Even though it tastes sweet, it has bitter and regretful effects. Try by all means to avoid it to the barest minimum.

Chapter 9

Is What You Are Eating, Eating You?

"And out of the ground the LORD God made every tree grow that is pleasant to the sight and good for food. The tree of life was also in the midst of the garden, and the tree of the knowledge of good and evil. And the LORD God commanded the man, saying, 'Of every tree of the garden you may freely eat, but of the tree of the knowledge of good and evil you shall not eat, for in the day that you eat of it you shall surely die.'" — Genesis 2:9, 16-17 (NKJV)

The foods we consume play a crucial role in our physical, mental, and spiritual well-being. They can either harm us or add life to our lives. They can either make us healthier or be the source of our illness.

Nutrition science has made significant advancements in understanding the intricate relationship between food and health. From the macronutrients of carbohydrates, proteins, and fats to the micronutrients of vitamins and minerals, each component plays a crucial role in supporting our body's functions.

Studies have revealed that the prevalence of chronic diseases such as obesity, diabetes, and heart disease has reached alarming levels in the world today and the major causes are poor dietary choices and excessive consumption of processed foods and sugars, which significantly contribute to these health concerns.

Embracing a lifestyle of wholeness is key. Building your immune system is crucial. You will not enjoy the abundant lifestyle without constantly strengthening it with a strong immune system. You can confess all you can but if you refuse to practice a healthy eating lifestyle, the words you speak will be of no effect in your life.

True nourishment extends beyond the physical realm to encompass our emotional, mental, and spiritual well-being. A lifestyle of wholeness integrates biblical wisdom, scientific knowledge, and mindful eating practices.

Through integrating Biblical Principles, scientific knowledge, and mindful lifestyle practices, we have the power to transform our health, elevate our consciousness, and align with the divine purpose of our existence.

The Power of What You are Eating

Have you ever heard the saying, "You are what you eat?" Now, let me bring to your attention another essential question: "Is what you are eating, eating you?" You might be asking yourself right now, "Does it matter what I eat?" I want to tell you that it does matter. If you have taken the time (or joy) to read this book to this extent, you should have settled in your heart by now that what you eat truly matters.

The Bible makes it clear in Genesis 2:9 and 2:16-17 that our food choices can lead to life or death. For instance, excessive consumption of sugar, which I referred to earlier as the "sweet killer." Yes, it is sweet, but the result can be lethal.

How many of us can be sure that we are not consuming foods that could lead to detrimental health effects? What about cancers? Consider cancers, for example—many cancers are significantly influenced by dietary choices. Are you certain that you are not inadvertently opening the door to diseases through your food choices? Think about this for a moment. Food is important to God; in the Old Testament, particularly in the book of Leviticus, He recommended, by way of commandments, a dietary plan for His covenant people.

God, who formed our bodies from dust, equally told us that the best food for our bodies comes from the earth. This is what He desires for us above all else. He cares that we eat foods that are the products of the earth—fruit-bearing trees, seed-bearing plants, herbs or vegetables, and clean meats. Foods that contain seeds promote abundant life (see Genesis 1:29 & Psalm 104:14). I believe God recognized their nutritional and medicinal value. Otherwise, He wouldn't recommend them for eating.

Jesus said in John 10:10 (NKJV), "The thief does not come except to steal, to kill, and to destroy. I have come that they may have life and that they may have it more abundantly." That is God's plan: life—not just for your spirit and soul, but also for your body. Do not give the devil any space in your life and health by making poor dietary choices.

God established His dietary plan at the foundation of the world and gave it to Adam in Eden. These same principles and simple guidelines have been passed down through Scripture to us. By taking a few moments to understand and adopt God's plan, we can be rewarded with health, happiness, and a more abundant life.

So, is what you are eating, eating you?

Prayer:

Lord, teach me what to eat, teach me how to eat, teach me to eat wisely, and help me to eat for Your glory. And as I eat, let my body be nourished to health, vitality, and wholeness.
In Jesus's name. Amen.

What Are You Feeding Your Spirit?

Jesus said in the Scripture, "'Man shall not live by bread (food) alone, but by every word that proceeds from the mouth of God.'"
(Matthew 4:4 NKJV)

We've discussed the importance of nourishing your body for radiant health. I also want to let you know that what you feed your spirit is equally important and may be even more crucial. Proverbs 18:14 (KJV) states, "The spirit of a man will sustain his infirmity; but a wounded spirit who can bear?" That is to tell you the importance and superiority of the human spirit. There are many instances where patients, given up by doctors and even by us nurses, have defied the odds because their faith and spirit sustained them. Their belief in their own healing helped them achieve victory and radiant health.

If you are a healthcare professional reading this book, remember this: we should not be too quick to give up on our patients. No matter how experienced we are in science, it is not our place to pronounce death prematurely. Let's create an atmosphere of life in their hospital rooms and speak words of encouragement and hope over them.

There is a level of spiritual strength at which sickness or disease cannot threaten your existence. When illness strikes, the Holy Spirit within you will raise a standard against it. Romans 8:11 (AMP) says, "And if the Spirit of Him who raised Jesus from the dead lives in you, He who raised Christ Jesus from the dead will also give life to your mortal bodies through His Spirit, who lives in you." This is profoundly true! Your spirit is the real you. It can sustain you through challenges, but only if you nourish it daily with the Word of God, which is the food of the spirit.

Another way to strengthen your spirit and build resistance to any disease is through the consistent practice of speaking in tongues (your heavenly language). As Brother Jude explains, "But ye, beloved, building up yourselves on your most holy faith, praying in the Holy Ghost." (Jude 1:20).

Did you hear that? You can build your spirit through speaking in tongues to the point where it becomes a fortress against sickness. Your faith in God's promises for divine health and healing will stand strong against any illness the devil tries to bring your way. However, you must feed your spirit with the right sustenance—specifically, the Word of God and speaking in tongues.

What victory would we experience if more of us understood the importance of studying the Word of God and praying in the Holy Spirit. As the wise king of Israel wrote in Proverbs 4:20–22 (New Living Translation): "Pay attention, my child, to what I say. Listen carefully. Don't lose sight of my words. Let them penetrate deep within your heart, for they bring life and radiant health to anyone who discovers their meaning." The Word of God, flowing from within you like rivers of living water, will fill your body with radiant health—it is life to those who find it and medicine to all their flesh, as said in the King James Version. So, what are you feeding your spirit? Is it the negativity from newspapers, television, and radio? Or the life that comes from the Word of God? The choice is up to you.

Prayer:

Lord, help me to order my priorities right, to put first things first. As I study Your Word, Lord, let me encounter the healing and health that is in Your Word. Help me to receive the life and vitality that is in the Word so that I can live a whole, healthy, and radiant life, in Jesus' name. Amen.

Chapter 10

The Power of Rest and Relaxation

"Come to me, all you who are weary and burdened, and I will give you rest. Take my yoke upon you and learn from me, for I am gentle and humble in heart, and you will find rest for your souls. For my yoke is easy and my burden is light." — Matthew 11:28-30 (NIV)

I remember all too well the feeling of burnout that crept into my life because of overwork and neglecting the need for adequate rest. It soon began to affect my health negatively until I had a rethink, strategize, and take adequate rest as and when due.

As leaders, we often overlook the importance of rest; we are only concerned about our goals and we are always ready to go the extra mile to achieve them even though it will cost us our rest time. Although it is good to be goal-driven and hardworking, we must also recognize that we are still human with a body that has a lot of limitations and often demands adequate rest from us.

This is where delegation becomes important. We need to understand that we cannot do it all; we must delegate tasks to trusted individuals around us. We must recognize the gifts in others, trust them, and hold them accountable to do what they are good at doing. Find the gift in them and let them soar and grow. Burnout and exhaustion will be at our door if we do not seek the help of others.

The scripture is clear about the importance of rest and rejuvenation. In the book of Exodus, God commands us to observe the Sabbath day and keep it holy. This divine directive serves as a reminder of the significance of rest in our lives, not just as a physical necessity but as a spiritual practice that allows us to recharge, refocus, and renew our energy for the journey ahead.

One of my mentors, John C. Maxwell, says it well: "Take time out of your busy schedule to just sit, relax, and think." Those are some of my best times away, just to think.

Jesus said in His Word:

"Come to me, all you who are heavy laden, and I will give you rest. Take my yoke upon you and learn from me, for I am meek and lowly in heart, and you will find rest for your souls." (Matthew 11:28-29).

The desire of God is not for us to work all day long without resting. The Bible reveals in Psalms 127:2, "It is vain for you to rise up early, to sit up late, to eat the bread of sorrows: For so he giveth his beloved sleep." From this scripture, it is evident that if you are still toiling and struggling without enough time for yourself and your family to relax and enjoy, then you are not yet walking in the complete will of God and haven't experienced the total love of God yet, even though He loves you with an everlasting love. An evidence of God's love in your life is that you enjoy rest all around you.

Chapter 11

Be Mentally Whole

"Beloved, I pray that you may prosper in all things and be in health, just as your soul prospers." — 3 John 1:2

When we talk about maintaining a healthy lifestyle, we often focus on physical health over mental well-being. But it is essential to recognize the interconnections between our mind, body, and spirit in achieving true wholeness. It is crucial to cultivate mental wellness by establishing healthy boundaries, nurturing relationships, and embracing the healing power of laughter.

Relationships are the cornerstone of our emotional and mental well-being, providing us with support, love, and connection. However, it is equally important to maintain healthy boundaries in our relationships to protect our mental health and preserve our sense of self. Setting clear boundaries allows us to communicate our needs, establish mutual respect, and create a safe space for authentic connections with others.

Practical steps to maintain healthy boundaries include:

1. Communicate openly and honestly with others about your needs and boundaries.

2. Learn to say no without guilt or shame when your boundaries are being crossed.

3. Take time for self-care and prioritize your own well-being.

4. Surround yourself with positive and supportive individuals who respect your boundaries.

Laughter is a powerful tool for promoting mental wellness, reducing stress, and fostering an atmosphere of joy and positivity. Incorporating laughter into your daily life can help you cope with challenges, enhance your mood, and strengthen your mental resilience. Whether through humor, playfulness, or shared moments of joy with loved ones, laughter has the power to uplift your spirits and cultivate a sense of inner peace and contentment.

Practical ways to incorporate laughter into your daily routine include:

1. Watch a comedy show or movie that brings a smile to your face.

2. Spend time with friends and family who share your sense of humor.

3. Engage in playful activities that spark joy and laughter, such as games, jokes, or creative pursuits.

4. Practice gratitude and find humor in everyday situations to lighten your perspective and foster a positive mindset.

Mental wellness is a holistic journey that encompasses the emotional, psychological, and spiritual aspects of our being. By prioritizing self-care, seeking support when needed, and cultivating healthy habits that nurture your mind, body, and spirit, you can achieve a state of mental wholeness that promotes balance, resilience, and inner peace.

Practical strategies for enhancing mental wellness include:

1. Practice meditation (upon God's Word) to quiet the mind and cultivate inner peace.
   Joshua 1:8 clearly states, "This book of the Law shall not depart from your mouth. You must meditate on it day and

night, so that you may be careful to do everything written in it. Then you will be prosperous and successful." This clearly means we will be healthy and whole.

2. Engage in regular physical activity to boost mood, reduce stress, and enhance mental clarity.
3. Seek professional help or counseling if you are struggling with mental health challenges.
4. Connect with a supportive community or network of peers who share your values and interests.

Bear in mind that self-care is not selfish but a necessary investment in your overall well-being. You need to prioritize yourself above any other person or thing and not feel guilty about it. You are only relevant on the earth because you are healthy; don't toy with your well-being.

Chapter 12

Radiant Health "I Am Factor"

"Nourish your body, mind, and soul with positivity and love, for a healthy 'I am' is the key to a fulfilling life." — Eva M. Francis

There is power in the words you speak into your life. You are the greatest prophet over your life and whatever you speak will surely come to pass. Therefore, I encourage you to speak God's precious words continuously over your life, making it a daily habitual practice. I want you to know that the tongue was not meant merely to speak but to send and release creative and healing words over your life. Declare God's Word daily, speaking it out loud enough for yourself to hear, and watch your life change as these words take effect. Remember, you are the number one prophet of your life.

1. I am the righteousness of God in Christ Jesus.

2. I am healthy, whole, and sound.

3. I am weighing the right weight.

4. I am an amazing person.

5. I am well today.

6. I am healed completely.

7. I am relieved of aches and pains.

8. I am eating healthily.

9. I am maintaining healthy blood pressure.

10. I am beautiful from the inside out.

11. I am happy and blessed to have strong bones and teeth, according to the Word of God.

12. I am enjoying my beautiful skin in Jesus' name.

13. I am not afraid of natural hormonal changes.

14. I am well-rested; I am not stressed.

15. I am at the right weight for my height.

16. I am healed by the stripes of Jesus.

17. I am whole spiritually, socially, and physically.

18. I am exercising adequately.

19. I am drinking plenty of fresh water to hydrate my body.

20. I am balanced in my life.

21. I am living a victorious life.

22. I am alert in my mind to everything God says in His Word about my healing and my health.

23. I am an energetic being.

24. I am eating wholesome food according to the Word of God.

25. I am healthy physically, mentally, emotionally, spiritually, hormonally, relationally, psychologically, socially, and corporately.

26. I am healthy in every organ, and every part of my body is healthy and made whole in Jesus' name.

A Prayer for Health and Healing

Father, in the name of Jesus Christ of Nazareth, I stand before You today declaring that health and healing belong to me. I decree and declare that every part of my body is healed and whole in the name of Jesus. I speak life over my entire body, for my body is the temple of the living God. I walk in divine health today, in Jesus' name. Today, my health is renewed.

In Your Word, You declared that those who wait upon You would mount up with wings like eagles, I claim that for my health today in the name of the Lord Jesus. I am strong and energetic, boldly carrying out God's plan and purpose for my life with a healthy body. Thank You, Father God, that I breathe healing and health into my life daily, in Jesus' name. According to God's Word, I confess with my mouth that Jesus is the Lord of my body and my life.

Healing Scriptures to Confess Daily

I have compiled below a daily dose of healing scriptures and confessions—God's medicine. Speak these scriptures and confessions over yourself each day. Meditate on them. Ponder them in your heart. Use them in praise and worship to your Heavenly Father. Remember, His Word is medicine—bringing life and radiant health to all your flesh.

Please say these healing scriptures daily, just as you would take medicine (See: Romans 10:10 & Psalm 1:1-3). The list of healing scriptures I have put below has revolutionized my health and well-being. I genuinely believe in the power of God's spoken Word. We speak what we see, and I am convinced of that. I believe that the more we declare these words over our lives, the more we will see the manifestations of health, healing, and wholeness.

"If you will diligently hearken to the voice of the Lord your God and will do what is right in His sight, and will listen to and obey His commandments and keep all His statutes, I will put none of the diseases upon you which I brought upon the Egyptians, for I am the Lord who heals you."
—Exodus 15:26 (AMPC)

"You shall serve the Lord your God; He shall bless your bread and water, and I will take sickness from your midst."
—Exodus 23:25 (AMPC)

"And the Lord will take away from you all sickness, and none of the evil diseases of Egypt, which you knew, will He put upon you, but will lay them upon all who hate you."
—Deuteronomy 7:15 (AMPC)

"IF YOU will listen diligently to the voice of the Lord your God, being watchful to do all His commandments which I command you this day, the Lord your God will set you high above all the nations of the earth. And all these blessings shall come upon you and overtake you if you heed the voice of the Lord your God."
—Deuteronomy 28:1-2 (AMPC)

"I call heaven and earth to witness this day against you that I have set before you life and death, the blessings and the curses; therefore, choose life, that you and your descendants may live and may love the Lord your God, obey His voice and cling to Him. For He is your life and the length of your days, that you may dwell in the land which the Lord swore to give to your fathers, to Abraham, Isaac, and Jacob."

—Deuteronomy 30:19-20 (AMPC) *"Every single good promise that the LORD had given the nation of Israel came true."*

"Not one of all the good promises that the Lord had made to the house of Israel failed; all came to pass."
—Joshua 21:45 (GW)

"Blessed be the Lord, who has given rest to His people Israel, according to all that He promised. Not one word has failed of all His good promise, which He promised through Moses His servant."
—1 Kings 8:56 (AMPC)

"My covenant will I not break or profane, nor alter the thing that is gone out of My lips."
—Psalm 89:34 (AMPC)

"With long life will I satisfy him and show him My salvation."
—Psalm 91:16 (AMPC)

"Who forgives [every one of] all your iniquities, who heals [each one of] all your diseases."
—Psalm 103:3 (AMPC)

"He brought them forth also with silver and gold: and there was not one feeble person among their tribes."
—Psalm 105:37 (KJV)

"He sends forth His word and heals them and rescues them from the pit and destruction."
—Psalm 107:20 (AMPC)

"I shall not die but live and shall declare the works and recount the illustrious acts of the Lord."
—Psalm 118:17 (AMPC)

"Trust the LORD with all your heart and do not rely on your own understanding. In all your ways acknowledge him, and he will make your paths smooth."
—Proverbs 3:5-6 (GW)

"My son, attend to my words; consent and submit to my sayings. Let them not depart from your sight; keep them in the center of your heart. For they are life to those who find them, healing and health to all their flesh. Keep and guard your heart with all vigilance and above all that you guard, for out of it flow the springs of life."
—Proverbs 4:20-23 (AMPC)

"Fear not [there is nothing to fear], for I am with you; do not look around you in terror and be dismayed, for I am your God. I will strengthen and harden you to difficulties, yes, I will help you; yes, I will hold you up and retain you with My [victorious] right hand of rightness and justice. For I the Lord your God hold your right hand; I am the Lord, who says to you, Fear not; I will help you!"
—Isaiah 41:10, 13 (AMPC)

"I, even I, am He Who blots out and cancels your transgressions, for My own sake, and I will not remember your sins. Put Me in remembrance [remind Me of your merits]; let us plead and argue together. Set forth your case, that you may be justified (proved right)."
—Isaiah 43:25-26 (AMPC)

"Surely, He has borne our griefs (sicknesses, weaknesses and distresses) and carried our sorrows and pains [of punishment], yet we [ignorantly] considered Him stricken, smitten and afflicted by God [as if with leprosy]. But He was wounded for our transgressions, He was bruised for our guilt and iniquities; the chastisement [needful to obtain] peace and well-being for us was upon Him, and with the stripes [that wounded] Him we are healed and made whole."
—Isaiah 53:4-5 (AMPC)

"Then said the Lord to me, You have seen well, for I am alert and active, watching over My word to perform it."
—Jeremiah 1:12 (AMPC)

"For I will restore health to you and I will heal your wounds, says the Lord, because they have called you an outcast, saying, this is Zion, whom no one seeks after and for whom no one cares!"

Jeremiah 30:17 (AMPC)

"Behold, I will bring it health and cure and I will cure them and will reveal unto them the abundance of peace and truth."

Jeremiah 33:6 (KJV)

68

"My people are destroyed for lack of knowledge; because you [the priestly nation] have rejected knowledge, I will also reject you that you shall be no priest to Me; seeing you have forgotten the

law of your God, I will also forget your children."

Hosea 4:6 (AMPC)

"Beat your plowshares into swords and your pruning hooks into spears; let the weak say, I am strong [a warrior]!"

Joel 3:10 (AMPC)

"The Lord is good, a Strength and Stronghold in the day of trouble; He knows (recognizes, has knowledge of and understands) those who take refuge and trust in Him. What do you devise and [how mad is your attempt to] plot against the Lord? He will make a full end [of Nineveh]; affliction [which My people shall suffer from Assyria] shall not rise up the second time."

Nahum 1:7, 9 (AMPC)

"And behold, a leper came up to Him and, prostrating himself, worshiped Him, saying, Lord, if You are willing, you are able to cleanse me by curing me. And He reached out His hand and touched him, saying, I am willing; be cleansed by being cured. And instantly his leprosy was cured and cleansed."

Matthew 8:2-3 (AMPC)

"And thus, He fulfilled what was spoken by the prophet Isaiah, He Himself took [in order to carry away] our weaknesses and infirmities and bore away our diseases."

Matthew 8:17 (AMPC)

"Truly I tell you, whatever you forbid and declare to be improper and unlawful on earth must be what is already forbidden in heaven and whatever you permit and declare proper and lawful on earth must be what is already permitted in heaven. Again, I tell you, if two of you on earth agree (harmonize together, make a symphony together) about whatever [anything and everything] they may ask, it will come to pass and be done for them by My Father in heaven. For wherever two or three are gathered (drawn together as My followers) in (into) My name, there I Am in the midst of them."

Matthew 18:18-20 (AMPC)

"And Jesus answered them, Truly I say to you, if you have faith (a firm relying trust) and do not doubt, you will not only do what has been done to the fig tree, but even if you say to this mountain,

be taken up and cast into the sea, it will be done."

Matthew 21:21 (AMPC)

"Truly I tell you, whoever says to this mountain, be lifted up and thrown into the sea! and does not doubt at all in his heart but believes that what he says will take place, it will be done for him. For this reason, I am telling you, whatever you ask for in prayer, believe (trust and be confident) that it is granted to you and you will [get it]."

Mark 11:23-24 (AMPC)

"They will pick up serpents; and [even] if they drink anything deadly, it will not hurt them; they will lay their hands on the sick and they will get well."

Mark 16:18 (AMPC)

"Behold! I have given you authority and power to trample upon serpents and scorpions and [physical and mental strength and ability] over all the power that the enemy [possesses] and nothing shall in any way harm you."

- Luke 10:19 (AMPC)

"We know that God does not listen to sinners; but if anyone is God-fearing and a worshiper of Him and does His will, He listens to him."

John 9:31 (AMPC)

"The thief comes only in order to steal and kill and destroy. I came that they may have and enjoy life and have it in abundance (to the full, till it overflows)."

John 10:10 (AMPC)

"He did not weaken in faith when he considered the [utter] impotence of his own body, which was as good as dead because he was about a hundred years old, or [when he considered] the barrenness of Sarah's [deadened] womb. No unbelief or distrust made him waver (doubtingly question) concerning the promise of

71

God, but he grew strong and was empowered by faith as he gave praise and glory to God, fully satisfied and assured that God was able and mighty to keep His word and to do what He had promised."

Romans 4:19-21 (AMPC)

"And if the Spirit of Him Who raised up Jesus from the dead dwells in you, [then] He Who raised up Christ Jesus from the dead will also restore to life your mortal (short-lived, perishable) bodies through His Spirit Who dwells in you."

Romans 8:11 (AMPC)

"For as many as are the promises of God, they all find their Yes [answer] in Him [Christ]. For this reason, we also utter the Amen (so be it) to God through Him [in His Person and by His agency] to the glory of God."

2 Corinthians 1:20 (AMPC)

"For though we walk (live) in the flesh, we are not carrying on our warfare according to the flesh and using mere human weapons. For the weapons of our warfare are not physical [weapons of flesh and blood], but they are mighty before God for the overthrow and destruction of strongholds, [Inasmuch as we] refute arguments and theories and reasoning and every proud and lofty thing that sets itself up against the [true] knowledge of God; and we lead every thought and purpose away captive into the obedience of Christ (the Messiah, the Anointed One)."

2 Corinthians 10:3-5 (AMPC)

"Christ purchased our freedom [redeeming us] from the curse (doom) of the Law [and its condemnation] by [Himself] becoming a curse for us, for it is written [in the Scriptures], Cursed is everyone who hangs on a tree (is crucified)."

Galatians 3:13 (AMPC)

"In conclusion, be strong in the Lord [be empowered through your union with Him]; draw your strength from Him [that strength which His boundless might provide]. Put on God's whole armor [the armor of a heavy armed soldier which God supplies], that you may be able successfully to stand up against [all] the strategies and the deceits of the devil. For we are not wrestling with flesh and blood [contending only with physical opponents], but against the despotisms, against the powers, against [the master spirits who are] the world rulers of this present darkness, against the spirit forces of wickedness in the heavenly (supernatural) sphere. Therefore, put on God's complete armor, that you may be able to resist and stand your ground on the evil day [of danger] and, having done all [the crisis demands], to stand [firmly in your place]. Stand therefore [hold your ground], having tightened the belt of truth around your loins and having put on the breastplate of integrity and of moral rectitude and right standing with God, And having shod your feet in preparation [to face the enemy with the firm-footed stability, the promptness and the readiness produced by the good news] of the Gospel of peace. Lift up over all the [covering] shield of saving faith, upon which you can quench all the flaming missiles of the wicked [one]. And take the helmet of salvation and the sword that the Spirit wields, which is the Word of God."

Ephesians 6:10-17 (AMPC)

"And I am convinced and sure of this very thing, that He Who began a good work in you will continue until the day of Jesus Christ [right up to the time of His return], developing [that good work] and perfecting and bringing it to full completion in you."

Philippians 1:6 (AMPC)

"[Not in your own strength] for it is God Who is all the while effectually at work in you [energizing and creating in you the power and desire], both to will and to work for His good pleasure and satisfaction and delight."

Philippians 2:13 (AMPC)

"Do not fret or have any anxiety about anything, but in every circumstance and in everything, by prayer and petition (definite requests), with thanksgiving, continue to make your wants known to

God. And God's peace [shall be yours, that tranquil state of a soul assured of its salvation through Christ and so fearing nothing from God and being content with its earthly lot of whatever sort that is, that peace] which transcends all understanding shall garrison and mount guard over your hearts and minds in Christ Jesus. For the rest, brethren, whatever is true, whatever is worthy of reverence and is honorable and seemly, whatever is just, whatever is pure, whatever is lovely and lovable, whatever is kind and winsome and gracious, if there is any virtue and excellence, if there is anything worthy of praise, think on and weigh and take account of these things [fix your minds on them]."

Philippians 4:6-8 (AMPC)

"For God did not give us a spirit of timidity (of cowardice, of craven and cringing and fawning fear), but [He has given us a spirit] of power and of love and of calm and well-balanced mind and discipline and self-control."

2 Timothy 1:7 (AMPC)

"So let us seize and hold fast and retain without wavering the hope we cherish and confess and our acknowledgement of it, for He Who promised is reliable (sure) and faithful to His word. Not forsaking or neglecting to assemble together [as believers], as is the habit of some people, but admonishing (warning, urging and encouraging) one another and all the more faithfully as you see the day approaching."

Hebrews 10:23, 25 (AMPC)

"Do not, therefore, fling away your fearless confidence, for it carries a great and glorious compensation of reward."

Hebrews 10:35 (AMPC)

"Because of faith also Sarah herself received physical power to conceive a child, even when she was long past the age for it, because she considered [God] Who had given her the promise to be reliable and trustworthy and true to His word."

Hebrews 11:11 (AMPC)

"Jesus Christ (the Messiah) is [always] the same, yesterday, today, [yes] and forever (to the ages)."

Hebrews 13:8 (AMPC)

"If any of you is deficient in wisdom, let him ask of the giving God [Who gives] to everyone liberally and ungrudgingly, without reproaching or faultfinding and it will be given him."

James 1:5 (AMPC)

"But the wisdom from above is first of all pure (undefiled); then it is peace-loving, courteous (considerate, gentle). [It is willing to] yield to reason, full of compassion and good fruits; it is wholehearted and straightforward, impartial and unfeigned (free from doubts, wavering and insincerity)."

James 3:17 (AMPC)

"So be subject to God. Resist the devil [stand firm against him] and he will flee from you. Come close to God and He will come close to you. [Recognize that you are] sinners, get your soiled hands clean; [realize that you have been disloyal] wavering individuals with divided interests and purify your hearts [of your spiritual adultery]."

James 4:7-8 (AMPC)

"Is anyone among you sick? He should call in the church elders (the spiritual guides). And they should pray over him, anointing him with oil in the Lord's name. And the prayer [that is] of faith will save him who is sick and the Lord will restore him; and if he has committed sins, he will be forgiven."

James 5:14-15 (AMPC)

"He personally bore our sins in His [own] body on the tree [a] [as on an altar and offered Himself on it], that we might die (cease to exist) to sin and live to righteousness. By His wounds you have been healed."

1 Peter 2:24 (AMPC)

"Casting the whole of your care [all your anxieties, all your worries, all your concerns, once and for all] on Him, for He cares for you affectionately and cares about you watchfully. Be well balanced (temperate, sober of mind), be vigilant and cautious at all times; for that enemy of yours, the devil, roams around like a lion roaring [in fierce hunger], seeking someone to seize upon and devour. Withstand him; be firm in faith [against his onset— rooted, established, strong, immovable and determined], knowing that the same (identical) sufferings are appointed to your brotherhood (the whole body of Christians) throughout the world."

1 Peter 5:7-9 (AMPC)

"And, beloved, if our consciences (our hearts) do not accuse us [if they do not make us feel guilty and condemn us], we have confidence (complete assurance and boldness) before God and we receive from Him whatever we ask, because we [watchfully] obey His orders [observe His suggestions and injunctions, follow His plan for us] and [habitually] practice what is pleasing to Him."

1 John 3:21-22 (AMPC)

"And this is the confidence (the assurance, the privilege of boldness) which we have in Him: [we are sure] that if we ask anything (make any request) according to His will (in agreement with His own plan),

He listens to and hears us. And if (since) we [positively] know that He listens to us in whatever we ask, we also know [with settled and absolute knowledge] that we have [granted us as our present possessions] the requests made of Him."

1 John 5:14-15 (AMPC)

"Beloved, I pray that you may prosper in every way and [that your body] may keep well, even as [I know] your soul keeps well and prospers."

3 John 1:2 (AMPC)

"And they have overcome (conquered) him by means of the blood of the Lamb and by the utterance of their testimony, for they did not love and cling to life even when faced with death [holding their lives cheap till they had to die for their witnessing]."

Revelation 12:11 (AMPC)

■ ▬ ■ ▬ ■ ▬ ■ ▬ ■ ▬ ■ ▬ ■ ▬ ■ ■

The Word of God will save your life.

"My son, give attention to my words; Incline your ear to my sayings. Do not let them depart from your eyes; Keep them in the midst of your heart; For they are life to those who find them and health to all their flesh."

Proverbs 4:20-22 (NKJV)

God's Word will not fail.

"Not a word failed of any good thing which the LORD had spoken to the house of Israel. All came to pass."

Joshua 21:45 (NKJV)

God's will—healing—is working in you (your body) now.

"for it is God who works in you both to will and to do for His good pleasure."

Philippians 2:13 (NKJV)

The Spirit of Life is making your body alive.

"But if the Spirit of Him who raised Jesus from the dead dwells in you, He who raised Christ from the dead will also give life to your mortal bodies through His Spirit who dwells in you."

Roman 8:11 (NKJV)

God is for you.

"For all the promises of God in Him are yes and in Him Amen, to the glory of God through us."2 Corinthians 1:20 (NKJV)

It is God's will for you to be healed.

"And behold, a leper came and worshiped Him, saying, "Lord, if You are willing, you can make me clean." Then Jesus put out His hand and touched him, saying, "I am willing; be cleansed." Immediately his leprosy was cleansed."

Matthew 8:2-3 (NKJV)

Obey God's Word and be healed.

"If you diligently heed the voice of the Lord your God and do what is right in His sight, give ear to His commandments and keep all His statutes, I will put none of the diseases on you which I have brought on the Egyptians. For I am the Lord who heals you."

Exodus 15:26 (NKJV)

Serve the Lord and healing will be yours.

"So, you shall serve the Lord your God and He will bless your bread and your water. And I will take sickness away from the midst of you."

Exodus 23:25 (NKJV)

God takes all sickness away from you.

"And the Lord will take away from you all sickness and will afflict you with none of the terrible diseases of Egypt which you have known, but will lay them on all those who hate you."

Deuteronomy 7:15 (NKJV)

Obey all God's commandments and receive all his blessings.

"Bring all the tithes into the storehouse, that there may be food in My house and try Me now in this," Says the Lord of hosts, "If I will not open for you the windows of heaven and pour out for you such blessing That there will not be room enough to receive it."

Malachi 3:10 (NKJV)

One of God's benefits is healing.

"Bless the Lord, O my soul; And all that is within me, bless His holy name! Bless the Lord, O my soul and forget not all His benefits: Who forgives all your iniquities, who heals all your diseases, who redeems your life from destruction, who crowns you with loving kindness and tender mercies, who satisfies your mouth with good things, so that your youth is renewed like the eagle's."

Psalm 103:1-5 (NKJV)

God's Word is healing.

"He sent His word and healed them and delivered them from their destructions."

Psalm 107:20 (NKJV)

God wants you to live.

"I shall not die, but live and declare the works of the LORD."

Psalm 118:17 (NKJV)

Choose to live. Be a fighter!

"I call heaven and earth as witnesses today against you, that I have set before your life and death, blessing and cursing; therefore, choose life, that both you and your descendants may live."

Deuteronomy 30:19 (NKJV)

You will live a long life.

"With long life I will satisfy him and show him My salvation."

Psalm 91:16 (NKJV)

Jesus bore your sins and your sicknesses.

"But He was wounded for our transgressions, He was bruised for our iniquities; The chastisement for our peace was upon Him and by His stripes we are healed."

Isaiah 53:5 (NKJV)

God will restore your health.

"'For I will restore health to you and heal you of your wounds,' says the Lord, 'Because they called you an outcast saying: "This is Zion; No one seeks her."'

Jeremiah 30:17 (NKJV)

You can take authority over the sickness in your body.

"Assuredly, I say to you, whatever you bind on earth will be bound in heaven and whatever you loose on earth will be loosed in heaven."

Matthew 18:18 (NKJV)

Agree with someone for your healing.

"Again, I say to you that if two of you agree on earth concerning anything that they ask, it will be done for them by My Father in heaven."

Matthew 18:19 (NKJV)

What you say will make a difference.

"So, Jesus answered and said to them, "Have faith in God. For assuredly, I say to you, whoever says to this mountain, 'Be removed and be cast into the sea,' and does not doubt in his heart, but believes that those things he says will be done, he will have whatever he says."

Mark 11:22:23 (NKJV)

Believe and you will receive.

"Therefore, I say to you, whatever things you ask when you pray, believe that you receive them and you will have them."

Mark 11:24 (NKJV)

Plead your case to God.

"I, even I, am He who blots out your transgressions for My own sake; And I will not remember your sins. Put Me in remembrance; Let us contend together; State your case, that you may be acquitted."

Isaiah 43:25-26 (NKJV)

Have someone lay hands on you for healing.

"And these signs will follow those who believe: In My name they will cast out demons; they will speak with new tongues; they will take up serpents; and if they drink anything deadly, it will by no means hurt them; they will lay hands on the sick and they will recover."

Mark 16:17-18 (NKJV)

Worship God.

"Now we know that God does not hear sinners; but if anyone is a worshiper of God and does His will, He hears him."

John 9:31 (NKJV)

The devil wants to kill you; God wants to heal you.

"The thief does not come except to steal and to kill and to destroy. I have come that they may have life and that they may have it more abundantly."

John 10:10 (NKJV)

You are redeemed from the curse.

"Christ has redeemed us from the curse of the law, having become a curse for us (for it is written, "Cursed is everyone who hangs on a tree"), that the blessing of Abraham might come upon the Gentiles in Christ Jesus, that we might receive the promise of the Spirit through faith."

Galatians 3:13-14 (NKJV)

You will not waver in your faith.

"Let us hold fast the confession of our hope without wavering, for He who promised is faithful." - Hebrews 10:23 (NKJV)

You can have confidence in God and his Word.

"Therefore, do not cast away your confidence, which has great reward." Hebrews 10:35 (NKJV)

Finding Strength in God's Word

You can find strength in God and his Word. "Let the weak say, 'I am strong.'"

Joel 3:10 (NKJV)

Jesus Christ has never changed. What he did in the Bible, he will do for you today.

"Jesus Christ is the same yesterday, today and forever."

Hebrews 13:8 (NKJV)

God's highest wish is for you to be well.

"Beloved, I wish above all things that thou mayest prosper and be in health, even as thy soul prospered."

3 John 1:2 (NKJV)

Be anointed with oil by a Christian who believes in healing.

"Is anyone among you sick? Let him call for the elders of the church and let them pray over him, anointing him with oil in the name of the Lord. And the prayer of faith will save the sick and the Lord will raise him up. And if he has committed sins, he will be forgiven."

James 5:14-15 (NKJV)

Jesus has already paid the price for your healing.

"...who Himself bore our sins in His own body on the tree, that we, having died to sins, might live for righteousness by whose stripes you were healed."

1 Peter 2:24 (NKJV)

Be confident in your prayers.

"Now this is the confidence that we have in Him, that if we ask anything according to His will, He hears us. And if we know that He hears us, whatever we ask, we know that we have the petitions that we have asked of Him."

1 John 5:14-15 (NKJV)

God answers the prayers of those who keep his commandments.

"Beloved, if our heart does not condemn us, we have confidence toward God. And whatever we ask we receive from Him, because we keep His commandments and do those things that are pleasing in His sight."

1 John 3:21-22 (NKJV)

Fear is not of God. Rebuke it!

"For God has not given us a spirit of fear, but of power and of love and of a sound mind."

2 Timothy 1:7 (NKJV)

Cast down those thoughts and imaginations that don't line up with the Word of God.

"For the weapons of our warfare are not carnal but mighty in God for pulling down strongholds, casting down arguments and every high thing that exalts itself against the knowledge of God, bringing every thought into captivity to the obedience of Christ."

2 Corinthians 10:4-5 (NKJV)

Be strong in the Lord's power.

"Finally, my brethren, be strong in the Lord and in the power of His might. Put on the whole armor of God, that you may be able to stand against the wiles of the devil. For we do not wrestle against flesh and blood, but against principalities, against powers, against the rulers of the darkness of this age, against spiritual hosts of wickedness in the heavenly places. Therefore, take up the whole armor of God, that you may be able to withstand in the evil day and having done all, to stand. Stand therefore, having girded your waist with truth, having put on the breastplate of righteousness and having shod your feet with the preparation of the gospel of peace; above all, taking the shield of faith with which, you will be able to quench all the fiery

darts of the wicked one. And take the helmet of salvation and the sword of the Spirit, which is the word of God."

Ephesians 6:10-17 (NKJV)

Give testimony of your healing.

"And they overcame him by the blood of the Lamb and by the word of their testimony and they did not love their lives to the death."

Revelations 12:11 (NKJV)

Your sickness will leave and not come back again.

"What do you conspire against the Lord? He will make an utter end of it. Affliction will not rise up a second time."

Nahum 1:9 (NKJV)

Finally, it is God's divine will for us to live abundantly prosperous lives. He wants us to be well and whole. Consider this: one cannot reach their fullest potential without good health. God wants us to be in the best shape of our lives to fulfill our divine assignment. Health, healing and wellness are our birthright, and God wants us to enjoy brilliant health and wholeness. If you are experiencing any health challenges, know that God cares about you and is ready to relieve you of physical pain and sickness. Never stop believing and never stop declaring your health and healing. He loves you profoundly.

Conclusion

Health and wellness are a result of the right interconnectedness of our soul, body, and spirit. This book has armed you with practical strategies, biblical wisdom, and scientific knowledge for experiencing wholeness in your spirit, soul, and body. It is time you put what you have learned into use.

Regardless of your current health challenges, by embracing the wisdom of the Scriptures, seeking guidance from science, and nurturing your souls with love and compassion, you are on your way to total healing and restoration of sound health. Surely, there will be obstacles and challenges along the way but as you align your actions with your intentions and trust in the Holy Spirit, you can transcend limitations, overcome obstacles, and manifest a life of abundance and joy.

Remember, to live and enjoy the abundant life God has for us, you must understand and believe that there is power in:

- Lifestyle Changes
- The Science of Health
- Biblical Wisdom

About the Author

Eva M. Francis is a board-certified registered nurse, philanthropist, business consultant, award-winning leader, motivational speaker, certified coach and leadership trainer with the John Maxwell Team, and author of several books. With extensive experience in critical care and healthcare management, Eva has dedicated her career to improving patient outcomes, fostering compassionate care, and leading individuals and teams. She has been instrumental in launching innovative communities and healthcare initiatives. Her commitment to excellence and passion for making a positive impact has earned her numerous accolades within the nursing and healthcare community.

Inspirational, visionary, compassionate, adaptable, collaborative, and accountable are just a few traits that describe Eva M. Francis. A former healthcare and hospital executive, she has successfully transformed organizational culture, resulting in improved hospital and departmental efficiency, multiple accreditations, and enhanced leadership development.

Eva M. Francis is results-oriented, with a proven track record of success in leading organizations toward improved business processes, effective clinical operations, patient care services, quality measures, and hospital operations, all contributing to enhanced bottom-line results.

Eva M. Francis is a transformational leader and strategic clinical program developer with experience in high-profile leadership and healthcare assignments. Beginning her career as a registered nurse in her native Jamaica, she migrated to the United States and completed her undergraduate and graduate degrees at Florida Atlantic University and Nova Southeastern University.

Eva M. Francis is a member of Words of Life Fellowship Church in North Miami Beach, under the pastorate of Pastor Geri Moore. "I want to recognize our late Pastor Stanley Moore Sr., under whose pastorate I sat for 28 years."

As a Critical Care Registered Nurse, Eva holds a Bachelor of Nursing degree and a Master of Science in Nursing Administration. She is the founder and CEO of Brilliant HealthCare, a healthcare training, leadership development, and consulting firm. Additionally, she is the founder and president of the National Nurse Empowerment & Leadership Institute, an organization dedicated to empowering, inspiring, and educating nurses and other healthcare professionals to succeed in their careers and businesses. Eva is passionate about Healthcare and Wellness empowered by Lifestyle, Science, Biblical Principles.

Eva is a former Associate Vice President of Nursing who served in Critical Care and Emergency Services at Mount Sinai Medical Center in Miami Beach . She has prayed for many of her patients and staff (at their request), resulting in manifestations of healing in their lives. An award-winning leader, Eva has extensive leadership training and experience. She has trained and mentored hundreds of healthcare professionals to advance and elevate their careers, particularly in leadership and business. Additionally, she has firsthand experience with the supernatural healing of an injured knee that physicians said would take three months to heal. By applying the Word of God to her situation and declaring her healing, she received her miracle and experienced a speedy recovery.

Eva strongly believes that the tongue should be used to release creative power consistently. The words that you speak will build your life or destroy it. "Let the words of my mouth and the meditation of my heart be acceptable in Your sight, O Lord, my rock and my redeemer." (Psalm 19:14 AMP)

To learn more or to speak to your team about Transformation Wellness or How to Live Well and Lead Well, connect with her at info@brillianthealthcaregroup.com.

Connect to her website: www.BrilliantHealthcaregroup.com

Other Books by the Author

1. A Guide to Nurse Entrepreneurship

2. 50 Business Ideas for Healthcare Professionals

3. Life in the Diaspora

4. 21 Principles

5. Get Well Lead Well

6. Leadership and Beyond

All books can be ordered from Amazon.

Made in the USA
Columbia, SC
18 February 2025

53840057R30059